A Challenge A Day
365 30-Day Challenges Ideas to Inspire, Motivate and Change Your Life

IMPORTANT NOTE TO READERS: This book has been written and published strictly for informational purposes, and in no way should be used as a substitute for consultation with health care professionals. You should not consider educational material herein to be the practice of medicine or to replace consultation with a physician or other medical practitioner. The author and publisher are providing you with information in this work so that you can have the knowledge and can choose, at your own risk, to act on that knowledge. The author and publisher also urge all readers to be aware of their health status and to consult health care professionals before beginning any health, diet, and/or exercise program.

This book is independently authored and published and no sponsorship or endorsement of this book by, and no affiliation with, any trademarked brands or other products mentioned within is claimed or suggested. All trademarks that appear in this book belong to their respective owners and are used here for informational purposes only. The authors and publisher encourage readers to patronize the quality brands and products mentioned in this book.

Contents

~~The End~~ **The Beginning of your 30 Day Challenge**

Introduction

Hi – I'm Anna – full time working Mom of two. I started experimenting with mini and 30-day challenges in 2015 in an effort to get my Son to spend more time being active and less time in front of video games.   After that, it was a 30-day challenge for my Husband to get in shape. Then it was a mini 14-day challenge for my daughter to get organized. It was then I realized that I live in a 75% competitive house. 2 out of the 4 of us are extremely competitive, 1 very competitive, and then myself, who is semi competitive. All 4 of us enjoy rewards for accomplishments. Throughout the process of designing several mini and 30-day challenges, it occurred to me that many others could benefit from this type of structured challenge to keep them on track. From fitness and nutrition challenges to learning how to play the guitar or becoming a better Mom, I've explored things that help me build better habits, get healthier, more productive, creative and inspired.

Since I began this journey, I've had many ups and downs but one thing remains consistent that the structure and regimen of a challenge has kept me on track time and time again, when I would have fallen "off track" and the sense of accomplishment that comes with completing a challenge has kept me inspired to continue with my self-improvement and motivational mindset.

Not all challenges have been successful, and not everything I've attempted has turned into a habit (although many have). But I have learned how to follow through on the things I set out to do – even when I didn't want to.

My hope is that my successes and failures can inspire you to make your own positive changes. And you can give yourself permission to explore and try things out and step out of our comfort zones, one day…or month… at a time.

Come and join me on this journey. If you haven't already, do sign up for the newsletter (it's free) and I'll send you a new 30-day Challenge Idea every day to keep you inspired and motivated! **Go to iChallengeHub.com/booknewsletter/ to get started today!**

THE POWER OF THE CHALLENGE

The Challenge is a powerful resource! **iChallengeHub** will provide you with ideas to help you explore the things that interest you, help build new behaviors, and create healthy habits that stick, in the form of mini and 30 day challenges.

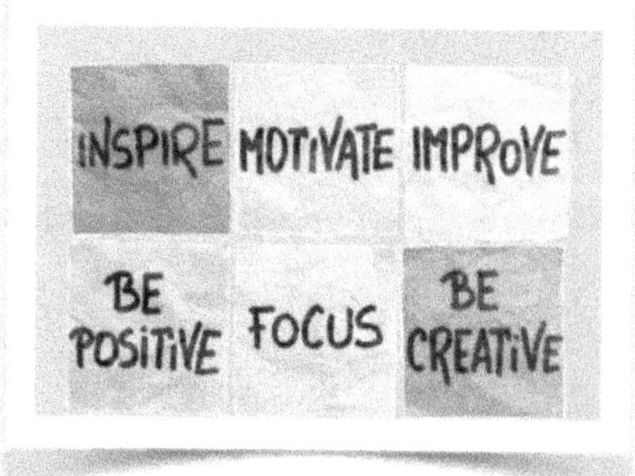

Mini Challenges motivate and inspire. A 30 day challenge is a proven strategy for implementing new healthy habits in life. They are powerful tools for change because they force you to do (or not do) one thing every single day, even if that something is small. People do all kinds of challenges, from fitness to food to health, self-improvement, learning, productivity, organization, relationships, personal finance, happiness and kindness, just to name a few. These challenges are designed to help you focus on the process of taking action every single day, because the consistency of action is what leads to change.

I've spent the past two years taking and making monthly challenges for myself and my family, in a quest to become healthier more productive and inspired. From learning to play the piano, to writing a book, to giving up sugar, my successes and failures have given me (and my family) a priceless education on the power of discipline, self-control, and the development of good habits. I've enjoyed the process immensely and have learned firsthand that continuous improvement and the commitment to investing in yourself pays dividends. This is why I keep taking on new challenges for myself and my family, and it's why you should give it a try as well.

What's your Challenge? *Find it here!*

HOW TO FOLLOW THROUGH ON A CHALLENGE

Challenges, whether it's a mini-challenge, or a 30 day challenge – any challenge begins and ends with commitment. A commitment to do something every single day, whether you want to or not. It's not an easy thing to do.

Over the years, through many challenges and countless hours spent studying the psychology of habits, willpower, and behavior change, it has been proven that a few key items can help you maximize your chances of success and to staying committed:

1. **Focus on one thing at a time.** Too many decisions are mentally exhausting, and will leave you frustrated if you try to keep it all up. So if you're taking on a health and fitness challenge, don't try to learn how to play the piano at the same time. Focus on health and fitness and nothing else.

2. **Plan it out and schedule it.** Decide what challenge you are going to do (fitness class),

decide where, when and for how long, and put it on the calendar. The more specific you can get about where, when, and how you will take action, the more likely you are to follow through.

3. **Make a public announcement.** Okay, well maybe not a press release, but a public commitment holds you accountable! So share your goal on Facebook, talk about it with friends, and participate in online communities.

4. **Reach out for help.** This can come in the form of books, apps, and websites that can help in areas where your skills are lacking. Don't be afraid to ask for help from people you trust and respect who can provide you with support and encouragement.

5. **Tweak your habitat.** Think ahead about how can you remove temptation and outsmart yourself so that bad decisions become harder to make? From putting your alarm clock on the other side of the room, to throwing out your junk food, to putting your workout clothes next to your bed. Whatever it

is...create an environment that makes it easy to stay committed to your challenge.

6. **Make contingency plans.** What will you do when you're not feeling well, traveling, going to a party, unmotivated, or having a bad day? Decide what kind of action you will take when you encounter the inevitable tough moments.

7. **Make it visual.** Photographs, inspirational quotes, your goal printed out in large letters, or a calendar with a checkbox next to every day that you've completed your challenge serve as constant and compelling reminders of what you're working toward.

8. **Track and measure your progress.** Tracking your results will help you stay focused, motivated, and more aware of what's working and what isn't.

9. **Don't quit.** If you mess up, don't quite. Learn from the experience and keep moving forward.

10. **Remove "I can't/I don't have" from your vocabulary.** This might be the most important tip of all. So many people underestimate how

much they can accomplish in a short amount of time. It's our nature to focus on why we can't and shouldn't do hard things.

- *I don't have time*
- *I can't write*

None of these should be part of your vocabulary. If you wait until you have all the tools and resources to do something, it will never happen. In order for us to grow, evolve and change, we have to do hard things. We can't avoid discomfort. Instead of telling yourself "I can't because…,"say "I can if…." The "if" forces you to change your mindset and focus on better, more constructive questions.

- *I can write workout if I wake up 30 minutes earlier every morning.*
- *I can learn the piano if I practice before I go to bed.*

Change is hard, but not impossible if you put a plan in place. But you <u>must</u> take the first step. Think about something you've wanted to change or try, give it a shot, and see what happens.

What's your Challenge? Get started today!

Before you start a 30-Day Challenges

A 30-day challenge isn't a lifetime commitment. 30 days is ideal for committing yourself to a daily challenge, because it's a long enough period of time for you to develop good habits and see progress, but short enough that it's not completely overwhelming or never ending.   Look at each month as an opportunity to start a new 30 day experiment. Whether you eliminate a bad habit or establish a healthier routine, you'll learn a lot about yourself and the strategies that can help you live your best life.

Sometimes, one simple change is all it takes to make life better. So start experimenting and challenge yourself to try something new each month.

A 30 day challenge can make a big difference in your life with a minimal investment. The majority of the 30 day challenge ideas that are in this book can be done anywhere — some of them for as little as five minutes a day, without spending any money or needing a ton of equipment.

Before you start any of the 30 day challenges, you can download and print any or all of the following resources from **https://iChallengeHub.com/bookresources/**:

- **iChallengeHub 12 month Planner** *(includes 12 30 day challenges)*

- **iChallengeHub Tracker** *(details of your 30 day challenge go here)*

- **iChallengeHub Calendar** *(document your daily steps here)*

- **iChallengeHub Accountability Tracker** *(who, what, where, when, how often go here)*

These are completely optional and you can start any of the challenges without them, but I find them useful to help stay on track, check off, and write daily notes to yourself to keep going.   Be creative and use them as an additional resource to stay motivated.

What can you achieve in 30 days?

A LOT! Which is why the 30 day challenge model has become so popular over the last few years.

30 days is plenty of time to create a new habit, learn a new skill or simply enjoy the sense of fulfillment that comes from challenging yourself to try something new.

There are 30 day challenges for almost every area of our lives from health and fitness to personal finance, so whatever your personal goals are there is bound to be a challenge to suit you! **<u>Get Started NOW!</u>**

How to use this book

You are encouraged to dip in and out of this book rather than read it from front to back, to find a challenge of interest to you.   The challenges are divided it up into 12 categories. If you are unsure where to start, you could begin by turning to a chapter you like the sound of and picking a challenge at random. As you progress with your 30 day challenge, I encourage you to use the resources in the previous page to record your progress, jot down any notes, along with any new ideas that spring to mind.

The 30-day challenges have been divided up into twelve main categories which you can access below.

- Food
- Fitness
- Health
- Learning
- Relationships
- Self-Improvement
- Organization
- Productivity
- Personal Finance
- Happiness
- Kindness
- Be the Best YOU!

How to get the most out of your 30 day challenge

> **Love the challenge**
> The biggest lesson that 30 day challenges have taught me, is to love the challenge. If you love to push yourself to try new things, build new habits and improve your life, the 30 day challenge is for you! They are a great way to try something new for month. At the end of the challenge, if you like it, keep going. If you don't, move on to something else.

> **Trust your intuition**
> Some of these challenges could change your life, others might be completely unsuitable for you — the idea is to use your intuition and find what feels right for you. I am not a medical physician, so if you are in any doubt as to whether a challenge is suitable for you, seek advice from your healthcare provider, doctor or those close to you.

> **Be resourceful**
> For me, resourcefulness is about looking around at what you have already and doing things. These challenges are designed to help you try new things in a resourceful and creative way, without spending a fortune to do so.

The ideas in this book are designed to give you inspiration, help you to start something new, or give you the opportunity to try something you've never done before.

Take a look at the challenges in this book, as a tool to help you to love the present moment for what it is. Who knows what new opportunities, inspiration and ideas might come out of your 30 day challenge! The only rule is: do something every day for 30 days. The rest is up to you.

Get Started Now!

Pick your 30 day challenge — do it every day for 30 days — love the journey and see what the future holds.

Chapter 1: Food

1. Drink More Water

It's the easiest and most natural thing to do. Whether it's 8 glasses a day or half your body weight in ounces, water gives us energy, flushes out toxins, promotes weight loss and is one of the easiest, cheapest, and best ways to stay healthy without having to give anything up. Add a fruit slice or sprig of mint for variety. Read more about the Drink More Water Challenge here.

2. Eliminate Sugar

Sugar is a carbohydrate that gives our bodies energy and provides fuel for our cells. It's made up of glucose, fructose (fruit sugar), sucrose (from cane or beet sugar), galactose, and other "-oses." In its natural state, fructose is rare, found mostly in seasonal fruits and some vegetables. In the early days of human life, sugar was scarce, and its presence triggered a reward center in the brain, making us genetically programmed to like it.

Food scientists and marketers have figured out ways to add sugar to practically everything, making our food cheap, delicious, and addicting. Due to the fact that sugar is a food that doesn't make us feel full, we eat more than we should. If not burned off, the sugar is stored as fat and can lead to weight gain, fatigue, obesity, brain fog, and cardiovascular issues.

For the next 30 days, eliminate all refined sugars along with artificial and natural sweeteners.

Anything that contains added sugar of any kind is off limits. Be sure to read labels, study ingredients, and look for anything that might be disguised as sugar, such as agave nectar, barley malt, cane juice, coconut palm sugar, dextrin, dextrose, fructose, molasses, and rice syrup.

Also watch out for foods that contain sugar, such as ketchup, barbecue sauce, sports drinks, applesauce, salad dressing, fruit yogurt, granola, soda, energy drinks, breakfast cereals, stevia, honey, maple syrup, and more.

CAN YOU EAT FRUIT?

Fresh fruit contains plenty of sugar in the form of fructose. If you make a fresh fruit smoothie, you can easily consume 35 grams of sugar. On the other hand,

3. Eat 7-9 Cups of Fruits and Veggies each Day

This food challenge is not about removing foods from your diet, but adding the right things to it.

The food we eat fuels the trillions of cells that live in the body with vitamins, minerals, and nutrients. They create the energy needed to keep the body functioning and protected against environmental toxins and other harmful things around us. Yet the majority of us don't consume nearly enough fruits and vegetables to keep our bodies functioning at an optimal level. I had to more than triple my daily vegetable intake, a task that proved far more challenging than I had anticipated! I realized that it's not enough to swear off bread and ice cream. We have to put the right things into our bodies.

For this challenge, eat 7 to 9 cups of fruits and vegetables every day. Vary the types of fruits and vegetables you eat, including:

- Leafy green vegetables, such as kale, collards, chard, spinach, and lettuce

- Colorful fruits and vegetables (the more colors, the better), such as berries, peaches, citrus, beets, and carrots

- Sulfur-rich vegetables, such as cabbage, broccoli, cauliflower, onions, garlic, mushrooms, and asparagus

- Make soups, purees, and smoothies. They're easier to consume, especially if you don't like the texture of vegetables. You can also use vegetable purees as sauces or toppings.

- Make a big, colorful chopped salad. I like to chop my leafy greens and colorful vegetables and mix them together in a large bowl. Over the next day or two, I'll grab handfuls of greens to either make a salad or a smoothie.

- Invest in a spiralizer and turn your vegetables into "noodles." From squash to zucchini, carrots to beets, the options are vast. You can also buy pre-spiralized veggies at Grocery Stores, Whole Foods Markets and now Birdseye offers them in the Frozen Food Section.

- Eat vegetables at breakfast. Whether you make a green smoothie, add spinach to your morning omelet, or add broccoli to your bacon and egg platter, you'll need to incorporate greens into every single meal.

- Eat your veggies first, then allow yourself to eat whatever else you want. Don't make the mistake of filling up with pasta or meat first.

Read: 19 ways to get your 9 servings per day here

4. Drink Hot Water with Lemon and Ginger first thing in the morning.

Drinking a glass every day can help strengthen your digestive system and prevent indigestion, nausea, and heartburn. I do this one every morning, and feel so much better for it. Drinking hot water feels so much better than cold water in the winter.

5. Drink Green Tea (high in antioxidants) every morning

I did this for a while and felt really healthy. You could see how you feel switching your regular tea or coffee for green tea. Remember green tea still has caffeine in unless you get the decaffeinated version

6. Plan your Meals

Once a week, (I prefer Sundays) set aside 15-20 minutes to plan your meals and grocery list for the next seven days. It's even easier when you have dozens of apps and websites willing to help make meal planning easier such as CookSmarts, Plan to Eat or 100 Days of Real Food.

7. Eat a Healthy Breakfast Every Morning

Eat a good, healthy breakfast every single morning. Nutrition experts have said that a healthy breakfast is a key start to the day. Not only do we perform better on the job and at school, but it supports our well-being in many other ways. A basic formula of good carbs and protein gives your body energy to get started and your brain the fuel it needs to take on the day! Click here for breakfast suggestions what to eat and what not to eat.

8. Make a Green Smoothie Every Morning

Start your day off with a green smoothie. It requires more planning, more chopping, more ingredients and, of course, a juicer or blender, but it's a great way to pack in some greens and fruits in the morning. I'm partial to smoothies because it incorporates all parts of the fruit and vegetables (where as juicers strip away a lot of the fiber and other vital nutrients). Find Green Smoothie recipes here.

9. Keep a Food Journal

Write down every single thing you eat and drink. Apps like MyFitnessPal (it has one of the largest food databases out there) are incredibly easy to use, or you can use a trusty pen and paper. Food journaling is said to be a powerful keystone habit, one that has a ripple effect into other areas of your life. Without realizing it, you just might find yourself eating better and exercising more.

10. Bring your Lunch to Work

Save money and eat healthier by bringing your own lunch to work. There usually are not a lot of healthy options readily available and the ones that are can be insanely expensive, or not that tasty. 30 Tasty options from EatingWell

11. Go Vegetarian for 30 days

Cut out all animal products for a month – it will be a great way to discover lots of vegetable based recipes.

There will be quite a bit of planning needed (especially if you work outside the house), lots of salads but lots of opportunities to experiment. <u>Read more about the meat-free challenge here.</u>

12. Cook a New Recipe Every Day

If you love to cook and you're up for the challenge and planning, then this challenge could be fun for you. Looking for a new recipe every day? <u>Try these</u>.

13. Food Presentation

There's just something about eating healthy food that looks good or "adorable", as my daughter says. So be creative....layer your greek yogurt, berries and almonds in mason jars. The same goes for your Cobb salad. Layered ingredients just look so much yummier than throwing everything in a bowl together.

14. Don't Drink Caffeine after 12:00

If you have to drink caffeine, do it before noon. This goes without saying if you often have trouble sleeping. Find other things such as short bursts of exercise or drinking enough water, to boost energy levels.

15. Read Labels

This one is about becoming more aware of foods with misleading packaging such as drinks that look healthy but actually contain a crazy amount of sugar. If you do find any surprises, see what alternatives you can use that are healthier alternatives for you. Learn more about label reading here.

16. Swap Unhealthy Snacks for Healthy Ones

I look at snacking as an opportunity to take a short mental break from work, have a moment to myself, and refuel my body. Healthy snack alternatives are important because you want foods that will make you feel good for the rest of your day without weighing you down or leading to a sugar crash before your next meal. Healthy snacks that have a good blend of carbohydrates from fiber, healthy fat, and protein are digested more slowly and keep you feeling full and your energy up until your next meal. Try fruit and mixed nuts, or carrot sticks and hummus.

Of course fruits, vegetables, and proteins, whether in the form of meat or nuts, are always ideal snacks to have on hand in between meals. But sometimes you just want a *little* bit something more. <u>Here are 121 Easy & Delicious Snacks for every type of Snacker.</u>

17. Eat Double Rainbows

Make your meals colorful! In other words, aim to consume two servings of foods naturally colored red (e.g. raspberries or red Swiss chard), orange (e.g. mangoes or carrots), yellow (e.g. lemons or bell peppers), green (grapes or kale), blue/purple (blueberries or beets), and white (bananas or onions). Each of these pigments represents hundreds— or even thousands—of disease-fighting, immune-enhancing phytochemicals," explains Julieanna Hever, MS, RD, CPT, a plant-based dietitian and author of The Vegetarian Diet and The Complete Idiot's Guide to Plant-Based Nutrition.

18. Get More Omega-3s

Take little steps each day to get more omega-3s. More and more research shows that omega-3 fatty acids help to keep your heart and your brain healthy. Filling up on omega-3 fatty acids does a body good. These polyunsaturated fats, which play a crucial role in how your body's cells function, have been shown to reduce harmful inflammation that could lead to heart disease, decrease triglyceride levels and blood pressure, and prevent fatal heart arrhythmias. Your body can't produce omega-3s, though, so you've got to be diligent about making sure your diet provides them. The good news is the fatty acids hide in tons of foods, like beans, certain oils and veggies, and—as you probably know—seafood. Take a look at these favorite sources.

19. No Eating after 7:00 pm

Take the no-eating-after-7:00 pm challenge and you might even realize you wake up feeling so great you want to make it part of your normal routine. I love this as it really does help you to lose weight as late night eating is often unhealthy and can make it difficult to drop pounds.

20. Don't Eat Anything that Comes out of a Box

Shelf-stable foods are often high in the types of ingredients we actually want to avoid (sugar, saturated fats and sodium) because they are used to ensure the food will last a long time on the shelf. Not to mention that most of the remaining ingredients are highly-processed or full of preservatives. The best way to help yourself eat more fruits/veggies (and thus fiber) is to avoid these types of foods. Cooking at home is encouraged!

21. Use Smaller or Portion Plates

Use salad plates instead of your dinner plates and you'll be surprised how much less food you eat overall. Take it a step further and use a Portion Plate, such as Marianne's Plate which can be found on Amazon.

22. Load Up on Protein

Challenge yourself to eat three meals per day balanced with lean adequate protein, complex carbs, and healthy fats, along with two protein snacks (for women) or three protein snacks (for men). For a woman of average height, which in the United States is 5'4", it is recommended to consume 110–120 grams of protein per day. For a man of average height, (5'11), it is recommended to consume 130–140 grams of protein per day. Check out these 20 delicious high protein foods.

23. Dial Down the Booze

Okay, we know this one is no fun, but a study published in the American Journal of Nutrition showed that alcohol is one of the biggest drivers of excess food intake. Another study published in the journal Obesity has suggested that this may be because alcohol heightens our senses. Researchers found that women who'd received the equivalent of about two drinks in the form of an alcohol infusion ate 30 percent more food than those who'd received a placebo. We're not saying you have to go dry, but if you replace your booze with H20, you might be shocked at how different your jeans feel in a week or two!

24. Eat More Antioxidants

Instead of satisfying your sweet tooth with some refined sugar, turn to berries and enjoy a slimmer waistline in no time. Berries are loaded with antioxidants, which can help reduce inflammation throughout the body. Berries like strawberries, raspberries, blueberries, and blackberries are also loaded with resveratrol, which is an antioxidant pigment that has been linked to reductions in belly fat and a reduced risk of dementia, to boot. So add them to your greek yogurt, snack pack or lunch for a quick, healthy, satisfying addition.

25. No Bread unless it's Sprouted

While it's often assumed that bread is off-limits when you're trying to lose belly fat, the right bread may actually expedite the process. Switching to sprouted bread can help out carb-lovers eager to get their fix without going up a belt size, thanks to the inulin content of sprouted grains. The results of a study published in Nutrition & Metabolism reveal that pre-diabetic study subjects whose diets were supplemented with inulin shaved off more belly fat and total weight than those whose meal plans didn't pack this healthy prebiotic fiber.

26. Eat More Nuts

Sometimes, to whip your body into shape, you have to get a little nutty. While nuts are high in fat, it's that very fat that makes them such powerful weapons in the war against a ballooning belly. In fact, research from Reina Sofia University Hospital reveals that study participants who consumed a diet rich in monounsaturated fats, like those in nuts, over a 28-day period gained less belly fat than their saturated fat-consuming counterparts while improving their insulin sensitivity.

27. Keep Meals Simple

Delicious, healthy food doesn't have to contain a lot of ingredients. Keep your meal ingredients to a minimum—just be sure to include a source of whole grains, lean protein, and healthy fat at each meal. For example, veggies and shrimp stir fried in sesame oil over a bed of grilled veggies seems restaurant quality but can be whipped up faster than takeout.

28. Eat Slower

Put your fork or spoon down between every bite, and focus on the flavors and textures of your food. You will be able to taste your food better and you can practice mindfulness while you eat and hopefully enjoy your meal a whole lot more. Chewing your food properly may also help with digestion.

29. Eat at Home

The easiest way to cut processed foods out of your diet is to eat at home. When you make your own food from whole, natural ingredients, you know exactly what's in it and don't have to worry that you're ingesting a potentially toxic combination of hidden chemicals. It can be quick and simple to make meals at home that can last you all week. Need inspiration? You can find tons of easy and healthy recipes here.

30. Grow your Own (veggies)

If you love to garden, you can't get much healthier than your back yard! If you live in a climate that offers a limited growing season, use the few months to take advantage of fresh cucumbers, tomatoes, peppers, broccoli, squash and zucchini! There is nothing better than a tomato, cucumber salad fresh out of the garden! Don't want your own garden? Visit a Farmer's Market in your area for the freshest of produce!

Chapter 2: Fitness

31. 30 Days of Exercise

> "You should come for a run with us," a friend said to me at a party one evening.
> "Sounds fun! I'd love to start running again," I replied.
> "How about Saturday morning at 8:00?"
> "Oh Saturday? I don't know, I think my daughter has a…"

This was typical for me. I had been making excuses for months as to why I couldn't work out, which is sad because I used to love working out. I used to be so committed and strong. If I were on vacation, I would find a park, or some stairs. But since baby number two came along, exercise had become a chore and an afterthought. I put everyone else first and myself last. I decided then and there to toughen up and get moving… and I did.

For this Challenge, you must exercise every day for 30 days.

There are no time limits or intensity requirements, no rules on what type of workouts to do or where. There's no worrying about pounds lost or strength gained. Your only job is to show up so that the behavior of exercise becomes habitual.

HOW I REDISCOVERED THE FITNESS HABIT
If there are two things I know about myself it's this: First, I cannot trust myself to work out on my own. Second, if I don't put it on the calendar and schedule the time, I won't do it. Someone or something else will always take priority.

Also, I need other people to tell me what to do, and the only decision I'm responsible for is to show up. So I signed up for lunchtime classes, recruited friends to work out with me, and asked a friend to be my "accountability partner" for the month. These were key to staying on track.
In the end, I did run with a friend. I enjoyed it so much that I went back again, and again, and again. By the end of the month, I'd fallen into a routine of runs, yoga, and long, leisurely walks. I pushed myself and worked out hard, even when I didn't have to. Most importantly, I found myself reuniting with the endorphins and hooked once again.

<u>**TIPS**</u>

- **Plan seven days of workouts in advance**. Better yet, sign up for, prepay for classes, and put it on the calendar.

- **Write in on and share your Calendar.** If you must exercise on your own, write your workouts down and send them to a friend or trainer for approval.

- **Set financial stakes**. They are a great way to stay motivated! For my challenge, I created a commitment contract on StickK.com, where for four weeks, I had to exercise seven days per week, with my exercises refereed by my sister. If I missed a workout, I'd have to give $25 to the NRA, which I really didn't want to do.

- **Create a reward system**. Set milestone rewards after your first week and upon completion of the challenge. I found the best way to motivate my Son was for him to work towards something he really wanted at the end of the challenge. *Some call it bribery....I call it challenge completion reward!*

- **Make it fun**! Go for hikes and long walks, call a friend, or make it a family adventure!

Whatever your challenge is…..use the tools and resources you find here to give you inspiration, help you to start something new, or give you the opportunity to try something you've never done before.

32. Walk 10,000 Steps Each Day

Ok, so I thought I was above average: I worked out a few days per week, I am always on the run, and I have a husband and two kids who seem to take it as a personal insult if I sit down. I do appreciate the benefits of walking. So, when I committed to walking 10,000 steps per day, I thought it would be easy. It wasn't.

Aside from being a nice, round number, 10,000 steps are also about five miles of walking a day. It encourages overall health and consistent physical activity to offset some of the negative effects of all that time people spend sitting. The American Heart Association and others promote walking because it's an easy activity for all fitness levels and ages. Walking also helps reduce your risk of heart disease, obesity and many other health problems.

I learned that I sit — a lot. I sit all day at work, and I'm in good company, given that most Americans spend six to eight hours a day sitting. I had to adjust my day to make sure I sat far less.

Before starting this challenge, I figured out my average daily steps to see how much I would need to change. Most days I can reach 6,000 steps pretty easily, it turns out, but that means I had some work to do.

Getting Started

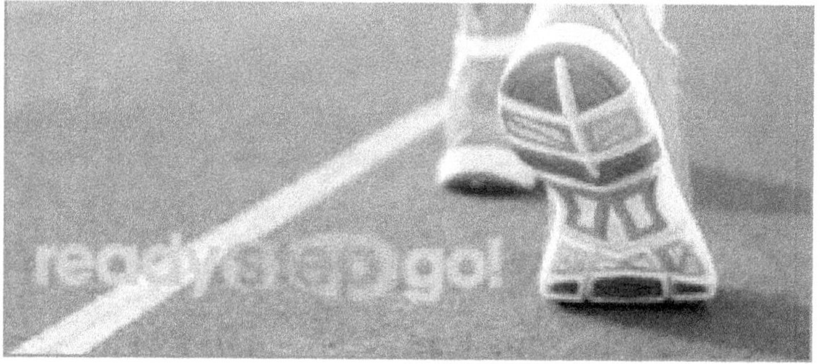

For some people, getting 10,000 steps may be easy. For others, going from a sedentary lifestyle to walking five miles a day can be tough. It's helpful to find your baseline of what you normally walk in a day.
When you know where you're starting, set incremental goals to reach 10,000. It's better to work your way up than to grow frustrated with a large goal and give up. Start by trying to get 4,000 steps a day for a week, and add 1,000 steps per day each week until you're doing 10,000.

This can be as simple as walking your dog an extra five or 10 minutes or parking at the back of your office parking lot and taking the stairs instead of the elevator. Adding in a brisk 10-minute walk three times a day is another great way to become more active. It also helps to set incremental goals for yourself throughout the day like I did by shooting for a certain step count by the time my kids left for school.

With that said we have a simple routine that you can build on, to make you stronger and fitter at your own pace.   The goal is to get up to 10K minimum steps per day.

To help you keep motivated and stay on top of your progress towards your goal of 30 days to 10000 steps, you can either:

1. Download a pedometer app on your Android of iPhone or
2. Purchase a **Fitbit.**
3. Download this printable **30 Day Walking Challenge**

Think of ways to get more steps in – park further, take the stairs, or take a break to run around outdoors with the little ones.

I decided to use a **FitBit Charge 3** to track my steps. The band lit up for every 2,000 steps and buzzed when I hit 10,000. The challenge of trying to get the band to light up and feel the final buzz motivated me throughout the day.

I aimed to have 2,000 steps before I sat down to work. Between getting the kids ready for school and walking to the bus stop, this was pretty easy. I also committed to taking a break every hour for five minutes or more to do something active, such as walking around the house, running in place or doing jumping jacks.

Then, I added in a 30- or 60-minute workout at some point during the day, whether it was a class at the gym, a jog around the neighborhood or 30 minutes on a treadmill. Most days I also did a short two-minute jog in place and some light stretching before bed, hitting my step goal around 9 p.m.

Reap the Benefits

I admit that on a few days I fell short. Still, I did see noticeable benefits from making the effort and hitting the 10,000-step goal most days.

- Better sleep: Running in place in the evening helped me relax, get tired and loosen any stiffness from sitting and watching TV before bed. I fell asleep easier and slept through the night.

- Heightened awareness: Aiming for 10,000 was an eye-opener. I didn't realize how much time I spend sitting. Now that I'm aware, I take more breaks and add in modest exercises throughout my workday.

- More energy: As part of this awareness, I get up and walk when I start to crash around 2 p.m. Rather than give in to moments of tiredness, I get moving, which has increased my energy. Taking walking breaks during the day also enhanced my focus while working.

- Shared motivation: Increasing activity didn't just benefit me but my whole family. The kids and I often stayed outside after school walking or biking rather than heading inside to watch TV or play video games. We went to parks and walked nature trails. It's easy to sleep in late or be lazy, but knowing I had a step goal gave me the push needed to stay active.

The Results Are In

Taking a step challenge is an easy way for anyone of any fitness level to become more active. You may be surprised to realize how much (or how little) you get up and move during the day. You also never know what accomplishing a step goal can do for your motivation — I'm continuing to increase my step count and working my way up to running a 5k in the next 30 days. Start simple and reach for the stars in 30 days or less!

33. Stretch Every Day

As you age, stretching continues to be important, even if you're less active. Your joints become less flexible over time. Inflexibility puts a crimp in daily acts, making it harder to walk, raise your arms overhead, or turn your head while backing up the car. It undermines balance, too, which can cause life-altering falls.

As with all types of exercise, you need to engage in stretching regularly in order to reap lasting benefits. If you only stretch occasionally, the effects are short lived. One study found that the greatest increase in hamstring length occurred right after the stretch and began to diminish within 15 seconds, though there was a noticeable effect for up to 24 hours. A daily regimen will deliver the greatest gains, but typically, you can expect lasting improvement in flexibility if you stretch at least two or three times a week.

A proper stretching routine of only 10 to 15 minutes offers many benefits, including increased range of motion, improved athletic performance, and decreased risk of injury and pain.

With this challenge, you will stretch EVERY DAY for 10-15 minutes.

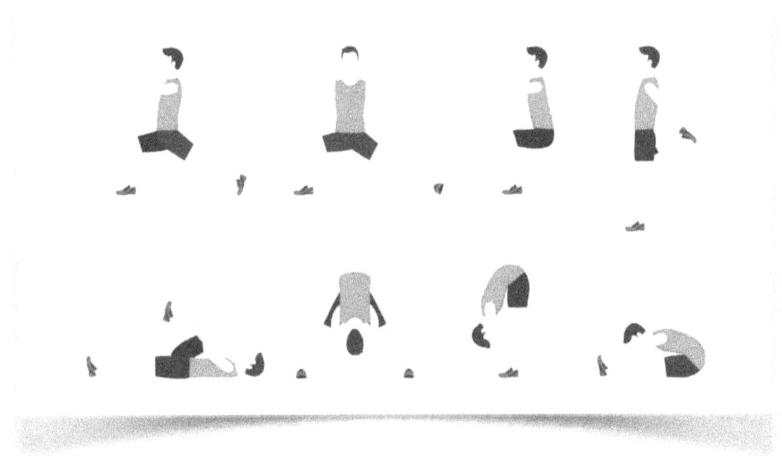

Hold each stretch for 60 to 90 seconds.

TIPS

- Decide where and when you'll stretch and aim to do it at the same time, in the same place, every day.

- Pair the stretching with another activity you enjoy. It will help pass the time, especially if you find stretching boring. For example, listen to music or an audiobook. Watch a television show or YouTube videos. Raise the stakes and allow yourself to do these enjoyable activities only while you are stretching.
- If you're looking to turn stretching into something meditative, focus on the spot in your muscle where you feel tension and breathe into it. Imagine your breath flowing into it while the muscles loosen up.

34. Do Yoga Every Day

People have been practicing yoga for thousands of years. This low-impact mind-body workout comes in many forms, styles, and levels of difficulty, and the benefits are vast. Beyond developing strong, toned muscles and improved flexibility and posture, yoga has the power to calm the mind and relieve stress. So it's time to grab your yoga mat and get started—your body and your mind will thank you for it.

Whether you sign up for a month-long package at a local yoga studio or practice at home with a video, commit to a 30-day yoga practice.

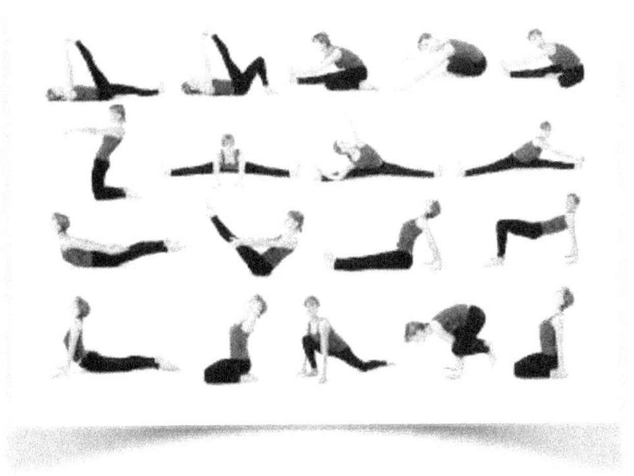

- Pay for group classes in advance, especially if you're the type of person who needs structure and accountability. Most local studios offer FREE trials. There are so many benefits to this.

- People motivate and encourage each other.

- You are much more likely to attend class when you make the decision in advance.

- If you know you'll be charged a penalty for missing class, you'll almost always show up.

35. Train for a 5K or Mini Marathon

Have you ever watched people cross the finish line of a local race and thought, "I could never do that?" Or are you an active walker, jogger, or runner who knows they can cross the finish line, but not sure on how to do it? With a little guidance and motivation, you can cross the finish line strong.

The 30-Days to Train for a 5K Challenge is the perfect tool to help you set your goal, work toward it, and reach it. Just follow this month-long training plan to help you get race-day ready.

Whether you're fitness newbie or gym rat, download this 30-day to 5K challenge to train for your first 5K.

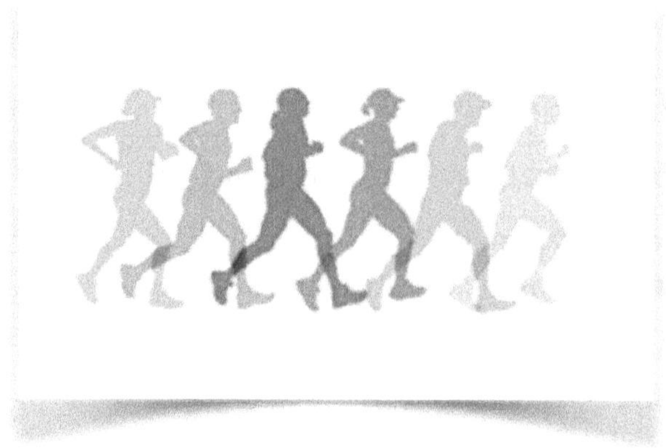

36. Dance Every Day

Here's the deal: I have known for a while that I need to up my cardio. I walk several times a week and am active but it's just not enough. I don't like running, some days walking sounds like a bore, and I'm not interested in going to a spinning class. It's been proven over and over that one of the keys to health and longevity is making sure we get a solid 30 minutes of cardio in several times a week. Bottom line: how can I get my cardio in and have fun at the same time?

I do however LOVE to dance. I'm not very good at it, but love it! Dancing is an awesome way to get that cardio in without feeling like it is boring old exercise.

It doesn't matter if you look like a fool. Put some music on and just dance freely for 10 minutes every day without caring what you look like. It's one of the most freeing things you can do!

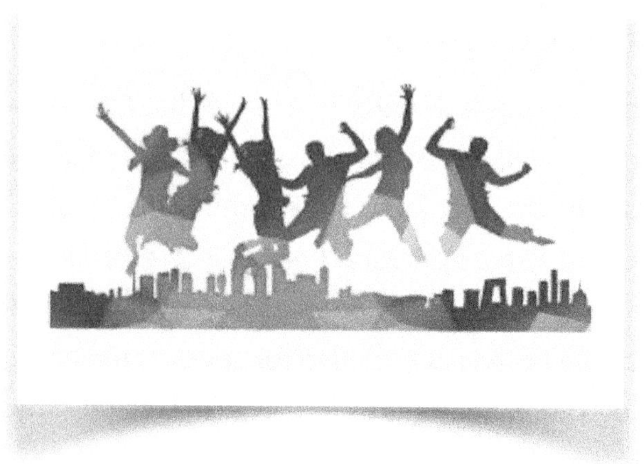

37. Take a 30 Minute Walk

There are so many benefits to talking a walk, besides
cardiovascular health. It helps mood, creativity, and
strengthens the brain. It's easy to do, you can go at your
own pace, listen to music, an audiobook or a podcast,
be outdoors (or on a treadmill watching television), or
with a friend.

38. Try a Home Workout

Decide how long you want your exercise routine to be,
find a workout schedule that's suitable for your level of
fitness, and get working out. Look for something that
works your whole body — you don't want to overwork

or strain a part of yourself by pushing yourself too much with just one thing. Try this Full Body Workout.

39. Bike

If you do this — seek out the best cycle paths and stay safe. Again, no guidelines. Just get on your bike and ride every day. Bike to work, bike around town or on trails. Find a cool cruizer here.

40. Take the Stairs

For 30 days, take the stairs. No elevator. No escalator. Stairs only.

41. Burpees

Burpees are an effective full body strength building and aerobic exercise, and very tiring and hard on the body. Work up to 30, 50 or even 100 every day. Check out the Burpee Challenge from Livestrong here.

42. Plank

Train to hold a 3 minute plank, a 5 minute plank (most common), or you can take the 30 day plank challenge. Try this Plank Challenge.

43. Pushups

Train to do <u>100 pushups in a row</u>.

44. Sit ups, Squats, Wall Sits

200 sit ups? 100 squats? A 2 minute wall sit? Pick a physical challenge that interests you and work up to your goal.

45. Whole Body Challenge

Focusing on one thing can be boring. Find a 30 day fitness challenge that incorporate lots of exercises for a full body workout. <u>Here is one you can try</u>.

46. Daily 30

Exercise for 30 minutes every day.

47. Incorporate Walking Meetings

Some meetings, like those in which you need to display a Powerpoint presentation, aren't conducive to walking -- but I'm willing to bet you can get creative, and find ways to transform other meetings into outdoor exercise.

For instance, perhaps you can transform your monthly brainstorming session into a brisk walk.

48. Walk Fido

Both Fido and the family will get the exercise they need. Have pre-teen children? Encourage them to start a dog-walking business to bring in a little extra spending money.

49. Play Tennis

Tennis is the perfect social sport for cooler evenings. Tennis is a good sport to maintain your health, fitness, strength and agility. **Tennis play uses nearly every muscle in the body. That includes your lower body, upper body, and core.** It has been calculated that an hour-long game of singles tennis burns around 600 calories for men and 420 calories for women.

50. Go Kayaking

Paddling a kayak helps to strengthen your "core" muscle groups, which are the major muscles of your trunk that move, support and stabilize your spine. The small, but constant muscle movements required to balance in a kayak, along with the rotational movement of paddling work together to build core strength.

With repeated paddling excursions, your core muscle groups will progressively strengthen—along with your abilities as a kayaker. Core conditioning also offers off-the-water benefits. For example, lifting a heavy object, reaching down or reaching up to a shelf all become easier when your core muscle groups are strong.

50. Go Paddle boarding

Paddle boarding improves core stability and balance whilst being as strenuous as you want to make it. It works your core and legs through the movement of bringing the paddle to the board.
Specifically, SUP engages the deltoids, rotator cuffs, traps, pects, latissimus dorsi, and your abdominal muscles.

51. Go Waterskiing

You don't have to be able to do 180s, flips and rolls to get a good workout when wake boarding. Beginners will discover that just getting up and traveling in a straight line requires a whole-body effort that will soon leave you feeling fatigued but invigorated. Here are a few of the health benefits of water skiing:

- Muscle Toning: There's a misconception that waterskiing is all about the lower body, but it's simply not true. It uses every muscle in your body. It develops your posture and your

shoulders and arms become quite strong
because you're getting pulled by your arms.

- Increased Balance and Core Strength: getting up
  on the skis- and staying up- require you to
  develop both your balance and core strength.

- Resistance Training: water skiing forces you to
  hold yourself up and keep going using resistance.
  It works core muscles, arm muscles, leg muscles,
  and all the muscles around them. It's also a lot
  safer that using free weights which can strain
  your muscles, and they don't even work the
  whole body.

- Easy on the Joints: Water skiing uses just about
  every muscle in the body without wearing down
  joints because it is all body weight resistance in
  free range of motion.

- Promotes strong legs: Tones up your legs fast.
  They absorb the energy of crossing the bumpy
  wake behind the boat, control your direction
  and are bent in a half-squat throughout, giving
  you particularly strong quads.

- Meditative aspect: Being on the water, much like
  in sailing, can have a calming effect on the mind

and forces you to focus on the task at hand, forgetting about the day to day stresses and worries. Not to mention that the endorphins from being active will keep you happy and healthy!

- Calorie burning: an hour session on water skis will burn about 400 calories.

- Good for Overall Health: As with all forms of physical exercise, water skiing can reduce or eliminate your risk for many health problems, such as high blood pressure, diabetes and obesity. It can also reduce your risk for coronary heart disease by reducing your triglyceride levels and increasing your "good" cholesterol.

52. Learn to Surf

Surfing is not as easy as it looks. It is worth taking some lessons to give you the basics and hopefully get you up on your feet.

As surfing involves the ocean, you should be a strong swimmer and always be aware of the safety aspects of being in the surf. If you are not sure about a suitable surfing spot, ask the local lifesavers or surf shop.

Having the right equipment is essential to get the best out of the surf. Your board should suit your body and your ability. For example, start with a long board as they are easier to stand up on, paddle and ride. Wear a wetsuit if necessary to keep you in the water long enough to learn.

Surfing provides many health benefits that we mentioned above, including:

- Cardiovascular fitness – from paddling

- Shoulder and back strength – these muscles will strengthen from the paddling

- Leg and core strength – once you're standing up on the board, strong legs and a strong core will keep you up.

53. Ski or Snowboard

Skiing and snowboarding are both great cardiovascular exercises that can help families burn some serious calories and lose weight.

- **Targets Lower Body** - Both Skiing and snowboarding heavily target the lower body muscles. Skiing naturally keeps the body in the squat position, which strengthens the quads, hamstrings, calves and glutes. Snowboarding also works some muscles that may not be used as often like the ankles and feet, which are engaged to help steer the board and maintain balance.

- **Improves Flexibility** - The very art of balancing and engaging the core and key muscle groups during skiing and snowboarding makes the body more flexible. It also helps to reduce muscle strains and sprains. Snowboarding especially improves flexibility tremendously as it requires the body to change directions frequently and swiftly.

- **Engages Core** - Keeping the body upright on skis or a snowboard requires some serious balancing skills and focus. It is not easy to stay steady on a slippery slope, while weaving down the trail. By having to constantly stay balanced, it forces the core muscles to work hard at engaging, which improves muscle tone in the abdomen and overall core strength.

54. Hiking

Hiking outdoors has plenty of perks: nice views, fresh air, and the sounds and smells of nature.

It's good for you, too. Hiking is a powerful cardio workout that can:

- Lower your risk of heart disease
- Improve your blood pressure and blood sugar levels
- Boost bone density, since walking is a weight-bearing exercise
- Build strength in your gluts, quadriceps, hamstrings, and the muscles in your hips and lower legs
- Strengthen your core
- Improve balance
- Help control your weight

Hiking is a great family activity. Use poles to make your upper body muscles work harder.

55. Do Pilates

Pilates is whole body fitness. Pilates improves flexibility, strengthens your core and improves your posture (less slouching can only be a good thing!). Pilates workouts promote strength and balanced muscle development as well as flexibility and increased the range of motion for the joints.

Attention to the core support and full-body fitness, including the breath and the mind, provide a level of integrative fitness that is hard to find elsewhere. It is also the reason that Pilates is so popular in rehab scenarios, as well as with athletes who find that Pilates is a great foundation for any kind of movement they do.

Pilates creates strength without bulk. Long, lean muscles are the name of the game here. In Pilates, you are not looking to build muscles for show. You are building toned muscles that work perfectly within the context of the body as a whole, and the <u>functional fitness</u> needs of a person as they move through life. One of the ways that Pilates creates long, strong muscles is by taking advantage of a type of muscle contraction called an eccentric contraction.

Other fitness benefits for Pilates are:

- Pilates Increases Flexibility

- Pilates Develops Core Strength

- Pilates Improves Posture

- Pilates Increases Energy

Just to name a few. If you are already active, Pilates will help lessen the risk of injury.

56. Try Rollerblading

Rollerblading was popular in the 90's and may seem outdated today, but it's still a great workout! It's a great mode of transportation over long distances- a good alternative to biking or skateboarding. Slimming, toning, endurance, balance, mood are just five of the benefits of rollerblading, just make sure that you wear a helmet, knee pads, and wrist guards!

Here are a few health benefits of rollerblading:

- **Increased Endurance**: in time, you can go for hours without getting fatigued. We recommend practicing 30 mins per day, in order to develop balance and reflexes and enjoying a feeling of freedom and lightness. In addition, rollerblading restores the suppleness of joints.

- **Improves Coordination**: Rollerblading takes a bit of practice in the beginning, but it improves flexibility and coordination. The activity forces you to even out your balance and find your center of gravity. Just like a consistent yoga practice, the more you rollerblade, the more graceful you will become during your everyday activities.

- **Great Cardio:** rollerblading increases the heart rate and gets your lungs working, both components in aerobic exercise. Rollerblading for 30 minutes at a steady pace raises the average heart rate to 148 beats each minute. It provides a cardio workout similar to running, and spinning. You can increase these aerobic benefits by skating on an uphill incline, skating more vigorously or practicing interval skating, which alternates one minute of brisk skating in a tucked stance with one minute of comfortable skating in an upright stance.

- **Good for Weight loss**: Thirty minutes of steady skating at a comfortable pace burns between 210 and 311 calories, while 30 minutes of interval skating burns up to 450 calories!

- **Firms the Lower Body:** The natural side-to-side motion your legs get from inline skating is ideal for trimming the thighs, strengthening the quads, and lifting the glutes. It's also a great low-impact aerobic activity that doesn't shock the joints.

- **Clears the Mind:** The swift and repetitive action of skating helps you stay present and gives your brain reprieve from constant noise. If you're skating in a quiet park, some music can help you get into the groove, but if you're out on the street, don't listen to loud music. Don't get so caught up that you're unaware of oncoming traffic.

57. Go for a Swim

Swimming is one of the best exercises you can do for all-round fitness. Being low impact, it is ideal for those who are currently injured or who have problems with high impact activities such as running. The range of swimming styles and strokes means that there is something for everyone, plus being in the water is also a good stress reliever as it forces you to focus on your breathing

58. Try Marital Arts

Martial arts can help you defend and protect yourself, but there are a number of health and fitness benefits associated with them as well.

There are several types of martial arts, including:

- **Karate**. This is the most common and well-known form of martial arts. Karate is a great way to tone and strengthen the upper body. In karate, an individual uses the hands, feet, and elbows for self-defense.

- **Tae kwon do**. Tae kwon do is related to karate, but focuses more on the legs and kicking, and less on the hands and upper body. Tae kwon do is good for strengthening and toning the lower body.

- **Judo.** In judo, you leverage the size and strength of the person you are fighting to defend yourself. Unlike other martial arts, judo focuses more on rolling and controlling opponents by holding them off, rather than by striking them.

- **Kung fu**. This high-intensity martial art provides a strong aerobic and cardiovascular workout. Kung fu involves primarily kicking and punching moves, somersaults, jumps, and evading an opponent. Kung fu particularly helps improve cardiovascular health.

Karate and other martial arts offer a number of physical and mental health benefits:

- **Conditioning.** The martial arts are a great way to tone and strengthen your muscles.

- **Flexibility and agility.** Practicing martial arts increases flexibility and agility, thereby improving your coordination skills.

- **Posture.** Good posture is beneficial for your health and can make you look and feel better.

- **Weight.** By burning calories and toning muscles, martial arts help you lose weight and maintain a healthy body weight.

- **Stamina.** Since martial arts provide a full-body workout, they increase overall stamina and endurance.

- **Mental health.** In addition to improving physical fitness, martial arts can improve mental and emotional health. As you learn self-defense moves, martial arts can give you greater self-confidence, reduce stress, and help you to concentrate and focus.

59. Try Horseback Riding

If you're looking for a non-traditional way to strengthen your core, horseback riding may be just the exercise you need. "Horseback riding really works the core muscles that stabilize the trunk: the abdominal, back, and pelvic muscles," explains Alison Stout, DO, of EvergreenHealth

Sport & Spine Care. "It's not just about the strength of the core, but the coordination and stability of it as well. The more you ride, the more the body learns to move with the horse."

Dr. Stout says horseback riding offers the following health benefits:

- **Core Strength**: "Horseback riding is an isometric exercise, which means it uses specific muscles to stay in certain positions, in this case, keeping balanced on the horse," Dr. Stout explains. "As a result, postural strength becomes very important in horseback riding."

- **Balance and Coordination:** "Staying balanced becomes more challenging the faster and more quickly the horse moves," she says. Cantering or galloping and jumping, for example, are much more difficult than a simple jog or trot. The rider must develop coordination skills to move the body with the horse in order to help the horse stay balanced.

- **Muscle Tone and Flexibility:** Along with the core muscles, the inner thighs and pelvic muscles get the biggest workout as a rider positions himself or herself. This exercise helps with good overall muscle tone and flexibility.

- **Cardiovascular Exercise:** Depending on the type of riding and the speed and agility of the horse, horseback riding can require more effort, energy, and cardiovascular capacity.

60. Shoot Some Hoops

Whether you are out shooting hoops by yourself, playing a game of pick-up basketball or on an elite competitive team, basketball is a great way to get fit and stay in shape. Here are a few reasons why playing basketball can help you stay in shape:

- Improve Motor Skills

- Strengthen Body

- Develop Mental Fitness

- Reduce Stress

- Burn Calories

Chapter 3: Health

61. Sleep for 7-8 Hours Every Night

Make it a priority to go to bed earlier every night and give your body the rest it deserves – you just have to find a way to allocate the hours. Need more reasons to take sleep more seriously? Read this.

62. Brush your Teeth Twice a Day

This challenge may seem easy and painless, but it is hard to do and do well. Dental hygiene is more important than we realize. Food particles in our mouths (especially from processed foods or foods high in sugar) can become a breeding ground for bacteria that impacts not just the health of our teeth, but potentially for the rest of the body as well.

63. Floss Daily

Work your way up to flossing (and flossing thoroughly) every day. You can start with just one tooth on the first day, and then work your way up to two, four, one side, then the other. Whatever gets you flossing. Once you get in the habit, it becomes second nature.

64. Take your Vitamins

Because we all have nutritional deficiencies (mine are iron, magnesium and vitamin D), especially if our diets aren't perfect.

65. Detox your House

Our houses are filled with toxic and synthetic chemicals. They're in our beauty products, household cleaning supplies, plastic toys, plastic cookware, dirty electricity and God knows what else. Over the next 30 days, slowly do a home makeover and replace your regular household items with organic, natural ones. Start with this primer on detoxifying your home, and also check out the extensive list of resources on the Environmental Working Group website and, for cosmetic and personal care products, the Think Dirty App.

66. Dress for Success

I often find myself falling into the habit of wearing a tank top, hoodie, and workout pants. Most days, I tie my hair back into a bun, dab on a little concealer, and head out the door. It's easy and comfortable. It makes my hectic life manageable. But at the same time, I don't like the fact that I don't put my own appearance at the top of the priority list. I enjoy dressing up. A great outfit makes me happy and I appreciate being complimented when I make the effort.

This challenge is for people who want to get out of the habit of throwing on the same outfit every day. For 30 days, get dressed every day. No workout clothes, loungewear, leggings, running shoes or flip flops allowed. Read more about the Dress for Success Challenge here!

67. Go to Bed at 10pm and Wake up at 6am

I've always felt really productive when I go to bed at 10pm and wake up at 6am. This is a good one if you often feel sluggish in the mornings or you never feel you have enough time to do everything.

68. Take a Nap

Extra sleep can help boost your memory, reduce stress and help you live longer. Naps boost alertness and improve motor performance, which is why you feel energized after one. The length of your nap determines the benefits. A 20-minute snooze—called a stage two nap—is ideal to enhance motor skills and attention, while an hour to 90 minutes of napping brings Rapid Eye Movement (REM) sleep, which helps make new connections in the brain and can aid in solving creative problems. Set an alarm to make sure you get just the right amount of sleep. (Napping for a length of time between 20 and 90 minutes may also help, but you're likely to feel groggy afterward.) The magic number for me seems to be about 45 minutes. For the Dos and Don't of napping read the Mayo Clinic's guidelines.

69. No Computer or Mobile Phone Screens after 7pm

We spend a large proportion of our waking lives connected to our phones, computers and other electronic devices. Try leaving the period before you go to bed or when it gets dark, technology free and see if your sleep improves. Some doctors believe exposure to blue light in the evening suppresses melatonin levels, and that people who are exposed to blue light before bed tend to not sleep as well. Read more about the dark side of the blue light from this Harvard article.

70. Go Snooze Free on your Alarm

As soon as your alarm sounds, hit the off button, take a stretch and climb straight out of bed, without wasting 20 minutes in snooze. If it's hard, set your alarm to a song instead. Looking for a "no snooze" alarm clock? Here you go!

71. Turn your Electronic Devices off Before Bed

Let's face it – electronics are a part of life. There is all sort of scientific evidence and words that I can't pronounce regarding the role of electronics, light and the science of sleep. Basically it comes down to this: If you sleep in a room with flashing lights and faint buzzing, it is common sense to say that you will have a more peaceful sleep if you turn your devices off. Read more about this from the experts at the Sleep Foundation, click here.

72. Place Lavender Under your Pillow

During my time living in the City, loud noises would often keep me up longer than usual, so I would place drops of Lavender on my pillow to help my sleep better. This, however, is not an old wives' tale. Some researchers have confirmed that when the scent of lavender is inhaled, it produces slight soothing, calming and sedative effects.

73. Get Yourself into a Bedtime Routine

Unwind properly before you go to bed and you could wake up the next day feeling so much more refreshed. Having a clear routine before you sleep might help, such as drinking a hot drink, cleansing your face, putting your pajamas on or reading. I don't have any research studies at my fingertips to back this one up, but it's worked for me as well as my kids when trying to get them to sleep.

74. Read Something that Makes you Feel Good Before you go to Sleep

I love reading before bed and feel that this isn't something that should stop at childhood. Even if you're not a regular reader, ask for recommendations and find a book or a collection of short stories you'll enjoy reading for a month. Here are six things that will happen if you read before bed.

75. No Complaining

Your iPhone crashes (again) and you want to throw the useless piece of crap out the window. Sure, it's therapeutic, but I've also come to realize how much complaining and criticizing we do on a daily basis. Negativity is everywhere and that kind of language and self talk affects us much more than we think. So instead of complaining (and using profanity, all of which are counterproductive) simply acknowledge the unfortunate situation and then come up with a solution. Read: **The 21 Day No Complaint Experiment**

76. No Devices in the Bedroom

If you're like me, your phone is probably the first thing

you look at in the morning an the last thing you look at before bed. All of this screen time may be eating away at our sleep.   Studies have shown that being exposed to the blue-and-white light given off by phones, laptops, and other electronic gadgets at night prevents our brains from releasing melatonin, a hormone that tells our bodies it's nighttime. That means it takes us longer to fall asleep. And many years of delaying sleep, researchers think, can mess with our internal body clocks. Some experts suggest not using our devices for roughly an hour before bed could help us fall asleep faster.

Your challenge is to keep the use of gadgets to a minimum and switch off an hour before your bedtime.

A few pieces of advice:

- Set your alarm an hour before bedtime to stop unnecessary scrolling on your phone and place your phone screen down on the floor to prevent notifications from tempting you

- Make sure that your bedroom is free of all other devices that emit blue light, including your TV and laptop. If you use a digital alarm clock, turn the face away from the bed to prevent the light from keeping you up.

77. No News

No reading or watching the news. If something newsworthy happens, let someone else tell you about it. The news can be addicting and depressing and just like the things we eat affect our physical health, the information we consume affects us mentally. I would imagine that after the first few days of "news withdrawals", the process would be quite liberating. And maybe at the end, you'll have a better process for consuming information in a more healthy and productive way.

78. No Social Media

I'm a social media junkie. I check it dozens of times a day, not because I care much about what other people or brands are doing. I do it out of habit. Imagine, then, how much I could accomplish if I didn't waste all those minutes on Facebook scrolling through the latest pics of someone's niece and nephew of which I have no clue who these people are!

79. No Shopping

Also known as the "stay away from Target" challenge. Decide at the beginning of the month what falls into the "acceptable" category and what items fall into the "off limits" category.

80. No Soda

I was Diet Soda junkie. Yup – 2-3 per day, every day.
This was not an easy challenge for me. Soda is a
stimulant. It is also addictive. And made up of all sorts of
artificial things which means that it has zero nutritional
value. Swap the soda for water and you will not only
save money, but you just might lose a few pounds too
(like these people).

81. No Snacking

We snack in the morning, we snack in the afternoon, we
pick on food when it's around even if we're not hungry.
And usually, it's not the healthiest of foods. If you're a
serial snacker (who favors the quick and easy), this is a
challenge for you. Taking out the snacks from our diets
forces us to eat more consciously during breakfast,
lunch and dinner.

82. No TV

There is so much great television out there and I'm a big
fan of unwinding with a show. But an hour or two of
television every night is an hour or two of time we could
spend doing other, more productive things.

83. No Caffeine

You may get headaches from the caffeine withdrawals,
so be prepared for the symptoms. Even better, reduce

your caffeine intake slowly in the week preceding your no caffeine month.

84. No Gossiping

Gossip is so much fun and so very tempting. Especially because it bonds us with other people. But gossip, in essence, is to speak "with the intent of eroding another person's reputation, image, or standing in the recipient's eyes". If you find yourself falling into the too much gossip trap, perhaps it's time to take a break from the negativity.

85. Don't Spread Yourself Too Thin

This is one of my weaknesses in that it can take me away from focusing solely on the most important thing, but at the same time, I get really enthusiastic and driven by trying new things. If you consistently spread your energy over too many things though, realize that multitasking may not be as efficient as you think it is and you could get a lot more done by focusing on one thing at a time.

86. Do Nothing for 30 Minutes a Day

If you're someone who finds it hard to switch off and relax, make a real effort to do nothing for a short period each day. We live in an illusion where we think the more we do, the more we'll get done, but we have to unwind sometimes too.

87. Spend Time in Nature or at Least Outdoors

Commit to spending a set amount of time outdoors each day, out in nature if possible. We underestimate how much being in nature impacts our mood. It has been said to reduce stress, improve creativity and general happiness. My favorite place is the peace and solitude that comes from sitting on my back deck listing to the birds and other relaxing nature sounds. There is nothing better than 30 minutes of relaxing time sitting, listening and observing. Just you and nature….

88. Learn to Love Yourself just a Little More Each Day

You deserve to treat yourself well. Be aware of negative self-talk and try to say and think kinder things instead. Hold yourself well. Do things that make you feel good and reflect on self-love for a month.

89. Practice Good Posture

Sit up straight and hold in your stomach when you walk. Keeping good posture will not only strengthen your core, but also add a small extra calorie burn because you're working slightly harder to maintain the position.

90. Wash your Hands

Wash your hands thoroughly with soap and water for 15 seconds frequently throughout the day and before you eat. Good hand hygiene helps prevent the spread of viruses and illness.

Chapter 4: Learning

91. Take a Photo every day

Take a photo of something that makes you happy, and something different every day. <u>Pinterest</u> has some excellent lists for a variety of different photography challenges.

92. Take a Video Clip every day

Record one second of video every day, or a clip of you dancing or singing or reading a poem, or whatever inspires you.

93. Word of the Day

Take a 30 day <u>vocabulary challenge</u> and learn the definition of a new word every day.

94. Read 20 pages every Day

After 30 days, you'll have read 600 pages, or two or three books! Where it can be overwhelming to say "I'm going to read three books this month", 20 pages per day seems so easy. So break it down into bite sized, daily chunks and set some realistic parameters around how much you want to read.

95. A Poem a Day Reading Challenge

Poems inspire and lead us to think about things we otherwise wouldn't think about. The Academy of American Poets features a new poem every day.

96. Watch a TED Talk every Day

They're usually less than 18 minutes long, which means that these speakers must put a lot of time and effort into conveying what's most important in a short amount of time. And there are some truly fascinating talks. Here are the most popular.

97. Read a Wikipedia Entry every Day

Set your homepage to Wikipedia's Random Page and learn something new every time you open your browser window. Or at least commit to reading one article once per day.

98. Learn (or brush up on) an Instrument

If you haven't touched a piano since high school, commit to practicing every day for 30 minutes. Or learn a new instrument. You'll be surprised at how much you can absorb with as little as 30 minutes of deliberate practice per day. And it's one of the best things you can do to strengthen your brain.

99. Learn a Language

Learning a foreign language is time consuming and incredibly frustrating, but it's important for brain health and it makes us smarter. And there are lots of <u>websites</u> that have simplified the art of language learning.

100. Learn a Skill

There must be something you've always wanted to try, like juggling, knitting, sewing, photography, drawing or dancing. Sign up for a local class or online and pick up a new skill. Need ideas? <u>Here are 101 New Skills to Learn to get you started</u>.

101. Learn to Cook

It's an important skill to have, especially if nutrition and fitness are important to you and, once you get over the fear of attempting to cook something, it can be quite fun. You don't need to cook full meals every day, as long as you cook *something.* Just start small, like boiling water and making pasta. Or you can take an <u>online cooking class</u> to learn the basics.

102. Write a Book

Some people write a 50,000 word novel in one month, as part of <u>National November Write a Novel</u>

Month (NaNoWriMo). Your novel will likely be quite terrible, but at least you can call yourself a novelist.

103. Write a Poem every day

There's also National Poetry Writing Month (NaPoWriMo), where aspiring poets attempt to write one poem every day for 30 days. How do you write poetry every day? Just start writing whatever's in your head. Spend 40 minutes or an hour and let your words dance.

104. Learn to Code

There are so many online programming classes available today.
From Codecademy to Coursera to Code.org to Khan Academy, these organizations has made learning to code easy and fun.

105. Memorize a deck of cards

It's a great party trick and an incredible memory training exercise. The free course at Memrise teaches you how to form associations between the group of cards and common characters to make the science of memorization easier. It's fascinating.

106. Start a Blog

It can be done with a lot of planning and hard work, one

that requires several hours or more of work every day. Prepare to brainstorm, research, write, write some more, design and promote – all in 30 days.

107. Make or Build Something

Build an app or a website. Knit a scarf, sew a dress, build a table, refinish a dresser, paint a picture, make a quilt. Find a project and just start get started.

108. Learn Photography

A criticism that is often heard today is that people spend too much time taking pictures of their experiences instead of living them. However, the photographs play the important role of allowing people to hold on to memories and show the rest of the world a peek into their lives while also telling a story.

Everyone should learn some photography because it provides several benefits. It is a fun hobby and can help you grow as a person by cultivating creativity.

In this photography masterclass, you can learn a complete guide to photography with 15 hours of training. It will teach you everything from understanding how your camera works to what gear you will need. It will also give you tips for selling your photographs.

109. Learn Self-Defense Basics

Nothing feels better than being confident that you can take care of yourself, whether it is mentally, financially, or physically. Being able to physically protect yourself in all situations is a reassurance that can only be gained through self-defense classes. While many people automatically think about women and children when they think about self-defense, it is really a skill for everyone. The key is to find your favorite martial art and learn some basic self-defense skills from a class in your area.

110. Learn how to be Funny

You're trapped on a desert island with two people. One is annoying, and one is funny. Just about everyone would prefer to be stuck with the guy with a good sense of humor, while leaving the annoying one back at camp.

The ability to be humorous is rooted in the ability to recognize absurdity, chance, circumstance, tonality, language choice and emphasis. These are all powerful skills independently, but together, they form the basis of humor.

When you are able to use humor effectively in writing, speech and socially. You will find yourself a sought after commodity, like the last piece of pizza after a college football game. <u>Learn how to think, write, speak and be funnier</u>

111. Learn How to Perform the Heimlich Maneuver

You're in the middle of a crowded restaurant and a man is choking on his chicken nugget. Not only is he embarrassed to be eating chicken nuggets, but he might die.

His only hope is that someone knows the Heimlich around him. The technique is simple, and anyone can learn it with a little bit of care and research.

This is a skill that every single adult should not only know but have practiced it until it is second nature. Learning this skill just might save a life. Learn: **<u>Choking: First Aid</u>**

112. Learn How to Perform CPR

CPR is another skill that every adult should not only learn but have practiced many times.

The time to learn this skill is not when it is your child or father needing CPR, but in your own free time.

CPR, or cardiopulmonary resuscitation, is the simple art of knowing how to jump start someone's heart and lungs with a little bit of your own air and chest compressions. This is an absolute must-have skill in emergency situations, and it's one of the first things that professional emergency medical transporters are taught.

It is also an easy skill to learn, but the potential payback is immense. Learning this new skill could easily keep a loved one alive until first responders arrive.

Learn here: <u>Cardiopulmonary resuscitation (CPR): First aid</u>

113. Confidence

Confidence is in recognizing your own strengths and living, breathing and speaking them. Confident people can have weak moments, but confidence is never weak. Self confidence is trusting in oneself. It is important to project confidence. <u>Here are 11 Habits to Nuture to Boost your Confidence.</u>

114. Positive Thinking

Life can be tough. Bad things happen to us all the time. Sometimes a past experience haunts us every day. It is easy to fill your mind with negative thoughts. But it is essential not to do this.

Positive thinking is a skill. It is something you need to work at intentionally to improve. Learning the skill of positivity is certainly worth the time invested.

When you have a positive mindset, you can take control of the way that you feel, behave and move forward, but you first need to start thinking in those positive, productive ways that provide energy rather than draining it. Read 100 Positive Thinking Exercises to Make Anyone Healthier & Happier.

115. Focus

Focus is the thinking skill that allows people to begin a task without procrastination and then maintain their attention and effort until the task is complete. Focus helps people pay attention in the midst of distractions and setbacks and to sustain the effort and energy needed to reach a goal.

If your mind is jumbled with other thoughts or busy trying to multi task your ability to focus greatly suffers. Like many mental and physical activities, focus can be increased and improved with effort. These 11 Exercises will Stengthen your Attention and Ability to Focus.

116. The Deliberate Practice Habit

Deliberate practice refers to a special type of practice that is purposeful and systematic. While regular practice might include mindless repetitions, deliberate practice requires focused attention and is conducted with the specific goal of improving performance.

Think about basketball. You have two guys practicing. Both spend one hour practicing. The first guy is running around doing a bit of everything. He does some jump shots. He practices dribbling. He chases after balls as they get away from him. He is not focused on his practice, he tries to do everything.

Now, guy number two is focused. He uses deliberate practice. He spends his hour practicing shooting from the key. He has a coach with him to catch his missed shots, gives advice on improving his shots and make sure there is little or no downtime.

The laser focus on a particular type of shot, means guy number two's practice will be FAR more effective than the same amount of practice time as the first guy.

This is the power of deliberate practice. Deliberate practice is a keystone habit. Once you learn to practice deliberately, everything you practice in life becomes easier to learn because you know how to build your skills the right way.
Read 8 Keys to Deliberate Practice.

117. Money Skills

Everyone likes to have money. They may not have a need to be rich, but it is certainly nice not to scramble to find creative ways to pay your bills.

However, money and finances are certainly skills, and unfortunately they are skills that most people have not learned.

There are skills in frugal living, budgeting, personal finances, debt management and reduction, saving, investing and more...

If you want to **learn a new skill**, and you don't know the skills of finance these would be a great place to start. They can help you make more money, spend less, keep more of what you make and even save money for investment, property or a future, "something special".

118. Stock Investing Skill

Whether you've inherited some money or you're saving money every month, you might be wondering about how you should invest your money to make it work for you. Learning how to invest your money is actually easier than a lot of people assume it is. You do not need to be an experienced trader to be successful in the stock market and in fact, it is often best to not move your money around very often.

While you may have heard that the best time to begin your investments was "yesterday," don't rush into making investment decisions that you don't really understand. Take your time to learn about the stock market, bonds, mutual funds, and trades. Once you learn the basics, you will have the confidence to put yourself on the right path. Read Investing 101 to find out how to make your money grow!

119. End Procrastination

Procrastination is the #1 business and life killer. We all procrastinate from time-to-time, but if procrastination actually keeps you from accomplishing important business or personal life tasks then this quickly becomes something that you MUST address.

If you want more info on why people procrastinate see these causes of procrastination. If you are looking for some quick-fix ideas on how to stop your procrastination tendencies see some methods for overcoming procrastination. But if you want to end procrastination once and forever, check out the link below, which I think of as the ultimate guide to fighting procrastination. Read this: *How to Stop Procrastinating:*

120. Stay Sharp

Keeping your skills active is the ultimate way to stay sharp. Anytime you walk away from something, you move further away from being able to do it at your best unless away time was sincerely needed. Keep at what you care about or you will be about as useful to achieving your goals as a dull saw is to wood.

Chapter 5: Relationships

121. Learn Something New Together

Spouse, child, friends are included here.   Sign up for a class or learn something new.

122. Read a book on how to improve your relationship in 30 days

Find a great book on how to improve your relationship with your significant other and read it from cover to cover in 30 days. You can even read it out loud to your partner.

123. Take the 30 day kiss hello and goodbye challenge

For the next 30 days, kiss your partner hello and goodbye. No exceptions! Make sure each kiss lasts for at least 5 seconds.

124. Take the 30 day appreciation challenge

Every day for the next 30 days actively look for something that you can praise or compliment your partner for. They'll feel appreciated and—after spending

30 days recognizing your partner's good qualities–you'll feel proud you managed to snag such a hottie!

125. Take the 30 days of surprises challenge

Have a small surprise ready for your significant other every day for 30-days. It doesn't have to be anything big. Surprises can include the following:

- Write a short love note on a post-it and leave it in their briefcase.

- Make a reservation at their favorite restaurant.

- Get a pint of that Ben & Jerry's flavor that they love.

126. Take the 30 days of questions challenge

Enhance communication in your relationship by putting together thirty questions you can ask each other to initiate interesting conversations. Here are some sample questions:

- What do you remember the most about our first date?

- What do you want for me to do differently when we argue?

- Let's plan a make-believe vacation: where would we go and what would we do?

127. Speak to someone new

It could be someone you've never spoken to at work, someone serving you at the bar or the person you're sitting next to on the bus.

128. Eat with people you care about

Can you sit down with people you love and eat one meal every day together for 30 days?

129. Be more assertive

This is something I've often struggled with and admire anyone who can get the balance right without sounding rude. For this one, think about people you know who do assertiveness really well and ask them for tips, or think about what it is that makes them assertive. You don't need to go out of your way looking for ways to assert yourself for this challenge — just set the intention to be more assertive and see where it takes you.

130. Strike up a conversation with a stranger while you're waiting for something

If you find yourself in queues quite a lot or you spend time waiting for something every day, seek out one person to talk with.

131. Befriend someone on the bus or train

My Grandmother talked about people she chatted with while she was on the bus. I don't see why we all shouldn't try this — even if it's just for a month. You never know who you might end up talking to.

132. Remember the names of new people

I've often been rubbish at remembering people's names but I'm getting better. Mentally repeating the person's name after you've been introduced helps, and so does associating that person with something. For example, on my yoga teacher training, my teacher Mimi managed to recall all 20 of our names instantly after asking us what our names were and our favorite food.

133. Improve your conversational skills

Sometimes I feel I'm better at expressing myself through writing, but give me the right conversation with the right people and I'm happy. This one isn't about reading some tried and tested formula — it's more about observing yourself when you're having conversations and improving in areas that make you feel uncomfortable. What do you mainly talk about with people? Are you mostly serious? When was the last time you made someone laugh? What can you do to improve your small talk or completely avoid it? Which conversations make you want to run away and why?

134. Eat together at the dinner table

I don't believe in any right or wrong way to eat, but if you never do this — give it a go for a month, even if it's just a few times a week. When you're in a family and you all have different interests, dinner time is often the place you can all sit and be together.

135. Listen more

Observe yourself when you talk with people. How often do you interrupt? Are you really listening or waiting for your moment to speak? What happens when you start talking less and listening more?

136. Spend time with people you like

This one might seem strange because why would you spend time with people you don't like, but I guess we do this one all the time. We stay in touch with people who put us down, we eat lunch with colleagues that irritate us, or we become a sounding board for people to offload. It might seem harmless, but people like this are energy drainers. Observe how many people are like this in your life and then re-evaluate who you spend the majority of your time with.

137. Understand Others' Motives

People might make passive aggressive comments when they're secretly feeling insecure, or react explosively when they need help. Rather than fighting fire with fire, seek to understand someone's behavior or motive for behaving in a certain way rather than lashing out.

138. Be selfless in your relationship

If you always have your own way and have started to take your partner for granted, treat him or her to this. The only rule is that you can't tell your partner what you're doing. So, for 30 days, be more selfless — make them tea, be grateful for little things they do, give more, listen more, be the one to stop arguments if it gets to that or do small gestures to make their life easier.

139. Give your partner space

I was given this advice by someone I teach meditation to. He said this helped his marriage a lot. When you give someone space, you allow them to be who they are. Whereas if you're too wrapped up in one another, there's a danger of losing part of your identity — especially if you stop doing the things you used to enjoy.

140. Be a good role model

You're already a role model for your child. Every time you say something, take an action or have a reaction to someone or something, your child is observing your behavior. While nobody expects you to be a "perfect" parent, it really isn't that complicated to raise happy, healthy, well-adjusted kids.

Kids need love. Kids need boundaries. Kids need someone to look up to and learn from.

Your job, as a parent, is to lead by example -- modeling the kind of behavior that you want your kids to adopt. Here are a few ways to lead by example, help your kids build character and self respect:

1. **Be your best**. When it comes to your kids, role-modeling is everything. Your children pay attention to everything you say and do, and they imitate your words and actions. Keep in mind how easily they are influenced. Be your best.

2. **Take care of yourself**. Being your best starts with taking good care of yourself -- getting enough sleep, making time to exercise, eating good food and finding healthy ways to manage negative emotions without lashing out.

3. **Be dependable**. You don't want to raise a kid who lets people down -- so make sure to model dependability.

4. **Be loyal**. We live in an era where removing a "friend" from your life can happen at the touch of a button. Show your child what true loyalty looks like -- showing up to help a friend in a time of need, or sticking with a local business owner who has served your family for years, instead of hopping over to the newest chain restaurant in your town.

5. **Be attentive**. As children get older, they push for more independence ("Mom, please don't come in my room!") and that's to be expected. But as a parent, your job isn't to be a "cool friend." Your job is to be a parent. Which means being attentive and making sure that your child isn't in harm's way -- even if your child thinks you're "annoying." *This includes knowing who they are with and where they are at all times.*

6. **Teach (healthy) skepticism**. Children are naturally trusting and they look eagerly to their surroundings for role models. Teach them that not all "role models" are reliable. Show them what it looks like to have a healthy skepticism and to "follow your instincts."

An example of this is a car dealership: "This man says that this is the best deal in town, but I have a hunch he might not be correct. Let's check out some other dealerships. It's important to trust your gut."

7. **Be accountable**. *F*ess up when you've done something wrong and don't make excuses. Take responsibility and admit that you did something unacceptable.

It's healthy for your child to see examples of grown-ups taking responsibility for their actions -- and enforcing "consequences" to correct inappropriate behavior.

8. **Enforce consequences** when your kid does something wrong. So many parents are hesitant to enforce consequences when a kid breaks a rule, but consistency is essential.

When your child does something unacceptable, you must implement an appropriate consequence. This is connected to lesson #3: Be dependable. Kids thrive on consistency and reliability. Without it, they invariably feel aimless and unsupported... and are at risk for developing into adults who don't know how to be consistent, either.

9. **Start now**. The habits that children develop at an early age tend to stick with them as they grow older. Since bad habits are tough to break, one of the best things you can do for your children, from day one, is to model behavior which positively shapes their character and values, and equips them to live responsible, productive lives.

>*The sooner, the better. The more consistent, the better.*

141. Be present

In our busy lives, we forget to slow down and experience the simple pleasures of life. Along with our many, many other jobs as parents, we have to model a healthy relationship with technology. We want to have a real relationship with our children so they can forge real relationships with others. If I don't teach my children how to connect with the human race, they may never learn how to have a successful relationship. Sitting around the Thanksgiving table with a bunch of iPhones just doesn't have the same affect, does it?

Here are a few tips on ways to form intimate relationships with people instead of dependent relationships on gadgets:

1. When you are with your children, be WITH them. Don't just put down your smartphone, put it away. Once it is out of site, it's less likely to distract you and shows your child that he is the priority.

2. Say out loud to your child, "I am going to do some work (schedule a dentist appointment, call a friend, etc.) in a bit on my cellphone, but right now I really want to spend some time with you. Tell me about your day."

3. Create boundaries around technology and apply the rules to everyone, including you and the other members of the household. If you've agreed to a no phones at the table rule or devices off by 9 p.m., it should apply to everyone, not just your children.

4. Teach your children the art of conversation by practicing with them. Ask open-ended questions of them and answer their questions to you thoughtfully and thoroughly. Skip the one-word

answers or the distracted "uh huh" when you are with them.

5. When you do, call them on their phone, set the expectation that they should answer or call you back. Too often phone calls receive a text in return. Why? Text is easier, safer, and less taxing than a phone conversation. But if your child is taking the easy way out of making a connection with you, imagine how difficult it will be for them to make a conversation with a stranger.

6. Keep private information private. What might seem cute or funny or endearing to you (Your 8-year-old son dressed up in his sister's dance costume! Your 3 year-old is finally potty trained! Your high schooler made the cheer team!) is not for public consumption. Show your child you respect him by using discretion at all times.

Most parents are hoping to instill a strong sense of self-esteem in their children. We want them to be capable, responsible, happy, healthy members of society. Sitting with heads buried in laptops or eyes scanning phones tells them that we think very little of them. We devalue them. Someday they will be gone and we will wish for more time with them. Save yourself the pain and be present now! This is when it counts!

142. Leave work at work

It is no secret that work can take over our lives. After all, we depend on our job to pay bills, feed our family, and create a better life. All too often we find ourselves being consumed by work, and this can cause discontent among family members.

Here are four tips to leave work at work:

1. **Make a To-Do list for the following day.** For many, it's the constant nagging of tomorrow's tasks or the fear of forgetting something important that keeps us from enjoying an evening (or weekend) away from the office. Rather than enjoying time with family or catching valuable shut eye, our minds are focused on the tasks that lie ahead... when we return to work.

2. **Disconnect from Technology.** Many of us have adapted the idea that we must be connected at all times. While it is harder to ignore work related emails outside of work, you can pick a few times at night to check your emails. You can

use inbox pause to hold your emails until you are ready for them.

3. **Don't dwell on your day**. There's a snowball effect that comes from dwelling on your problems and causes you to complain more. Use your evening commute home to reflect on your day and refocus your mind.

4. **Engage in humor**. In the end, laughter can be the best medicine. Laughter releases endorphins that lower stress and tension and mentally revive you. So listen to a podcast on your commute home, tune into Netflix for a comedy or <u>browse the top 20 funniest youtube videos.</u>

When you walk in the door at night, take a moment to remind yourself that you are not at work anymore. Let go of the day's distractions, or at the very least, make a conscious decision to put them off until later.

143. Start a tradition

Traditions offer numerous benefits to our families, including but not limited to the fact that they:

1. **Provide a source of identity**. Traditions and rituals often tell a story about a family.

Traditions can serve as reminders of events that have shaped your family and your children (e.g. every year your family rents the same lake house, and each time you go it reminds you of all the experiences you've had on previous trips).

2. **Strengthen the family bond.** Researchers have consistently found that families that engage in frequent traditions report stronger connection and unity than families that haven't established rituals together.

3. **Offer comfort and security**. Family traditions and rituals are the antidote to the harried feeling that comes from our fast-paced and ever-changing world. It's comforting to have a few constants in your life.

4. **Teach values.** One of the main purposes of rituals, whether religious or not, is to impart and reinforce values. The same goes with family traditions. Through daily family prayer, the importance of faith is re-enforced; through nightly bedtime stories, the value of education, reading, and life-long learning is inculcated; and through regular family dinners or activities, the family solidarity is instilled.

5. **Connects generations.** Family traditions are a
    great way to cultivate that valuable
    grandparental involvement. Growing up, our
    family would head to the Woods to spend
    weekends at my family's camp. I have lots of
    great memories fishing, swimming and riding dirt
    bikes with my cousins at my Grandparent's
    camp.

6. **Create lasting memories.** When kids are asked
    what they remember most about their
    childhood, most responded by talking about
    simple, everyday traditions like family dinners,
    holiday get-togethers, and bedtime stories.
    Those positive childhood memories can help
    make your child a happier and more generous
    adult.

144. De-clutter your schedule

If your schedule is a bit out of control and you are not
able to devote the time you would like to family and
friends, try these tips:

> 1. **Acknowledge the fact that you can't do
> everything**. We can only do so much. We have
> unlimited options, but limited resources. We
> have to make important decisions to eliminate

some things. When we're feeling especially productive and superhuman, we struggle to admit this reality. But, we can't do it all. We have to remove the clutter. Clutter is the stuff that interferes with the life we want to live. It slows us down from doing the things we value most. It's that unnecessary stuff that we entertain, but doesn't help us get where we want to go. And it needs to be removed.

2. Clarify what's most important…to you! The things that are important to you will affect how you make decisions and how you spend your days. If you don't know where you're going, why bother establishing a path? Before you start developing a plan, you have to know what you want to accomplish and what rules you will play by. You need a what and a why before you figure out how.

3. Determine what you have to do to live for those things. Once you've identified your objective, you can begin to think about how you'll get there. It is incredibly important to identify your goals and values. But if you don't take the second step and think about your plan to live up to them, then they are only dreams.

4. Say "no" to other stuff. It's not enough to know what things you should do. You also have to get clarity on the types of things you should not do. We've already established that our time is limited. We will have to make choices about how we spend our time. We will have say "no" to some things so we can say "yes" to others.

5. Find what motivates you and use it. Figure out what makes you tick. What makes you come alive? What makes you feel human and reminds you that you are not just a robot with a job and a checkbook? What tugs at your heart? What reminds you of the things you value most? It may be: listening to music, blogging, dancing, painting, singing, jogging, lifting weights, or something really random and strange that you just love to do.

Life is too short to spend our days in constant frustration.

Don't allow things of lesser importance to rob you of the life you could be living!

145. Be thankful

In our life, we sometimes spend too much time complaining about the things we do not like or even the things we have. Today and every day we need to take time to be thankful for the blessings we've been given.

146.   Go for a walk after dinner

After a long day, it is tempting to plop down on the couch after dinner and turn on Netflix or the TV. Don't do it! Do like the Italians do and go for a walk!

Called la passeggiata, the tradition of the after-dinner stroll isn't about getting their heart rate up or working off those carbs. It's about simply moseying around with loved ones—getting some fresh air, spending time with family, and stumbling into friends along the way, says Marie Spano, M.S., R.D., C.S.C.S., whose grandparents hail from Italy.

Compare that to most American families' post-dinner routines of watching TV, paying bills, or checking social media, and it's easy to see how going on a walk around the block immediately following dinner can help improve your family's health.

For time-strapped Americans, that's perhaps the best part of la passeggiata: It takes so little time. Even 10 to

15 minutes will have noticeable benefits. And the longer lease on life as well as valuable time spent with family is well worth the time investment.

147. Plan a gadget-free day

Technology has become such a ubiquitous part of our lives that some people actually exhibit signs of addictive withdrawal if they're away from their gadgets for too long.

Children in the US, ages 0 to 8, spend an average of 2 hours and 19 minutes a day with screen media. (Older kids spend even more time.)

While media and technology are important tools, helping nurture qualities like reverence, respect, curiosity, and creativity in our children (and ourselves) necessitates mindfully planning time to tap into the natural world and our creative selves.

- Take this small step: Plan a gadget-free day — with no TV, video games, computer, or other electronics — and relish finding creative, fun ways for your family to spend time together (preferably in a natural setting).

If you enjoy this special time (give it a few times before deciding), try to integrate it regularly into your week or month. You might consider not mentioning to your child(ren) that this is gadget-free day — simply plan a fun day without the influence of technology.

148. Take a family fitness class

Parents are unquestionably the number one influence in a child's life, acting as teachers, mentors, motivational coaches, and role models (among other things!). This is a huge responsibility. Children tend to watch their parents' every move, imitating their habits and actions.

So, if parents are sedentary, chances are their children will be as well. However, parents who eat a healthy diet and exercise on their own or with their children on a regular basis are teaching them some valuable lessons and setting a foundation for lifelong healthy living.

When parents promote fitness as an important family value, children are more likely to remain active throughout childhood – even as many of their peers turn to television shows and computer games.

Parents should practice what they preach if they want to make a healthy lifestyle a top priority in the lives of their children as they age. Taking a group fitness class offer multiple benefits, such as, fitness, health and quality family time.

149. Plan an adventure vacation

If you are seeking a memorable family trip, consider planning an adventure vacation!

A few benefits include:

- **Quality Family Time**. Adventure travel takes you to new places and the shared experience of it all brings you closer together as a family. When removed from your everyday setting, you'll learn more about each other and see your family members from a renewed perspective.

- **Natural Thrills**. Rafting on rapids, hiking among ancient ruins, biking next to a volcano... All of these activities are so much more exciting and natural than being at a theme park or on a cruise! Whether you are new to adventure travel or have done many trips before, adventure travel is exciting by nature. And who better to share this natural excitement with than your beloved family?

- **Learning Experiences**. The world becomes your classroom on an adventure trip. Whether you are young or old, there is always something to be learned from experiencing another culture, meeting new people and seeing life from a renewed perspective.

- **Encourages Health & Wellness**. Active vacations encourage the whole family to embrace an active lifestyle. Together, whatever your ages, you can discover the joys of hiking, biking, kayaking and more while on vacation, and maybe take some of this inspiration home with you too!

- **Amazing Memories.** A family vacation is meant to be memorable, above all else. By planning something beyond the standard family trip, and actively exploring somewhere new together, you'll create and share memories that will last a lifetime!

150. Sign up for a fun run or walk

Looking for a great way to get everyone moving? Sign up for a fun run or walk.

Think about all the benefits: Working together toward a common goal helps keep everyone motivated to move. When you move more, your family will feel better mentally and physically. That helps everyone avoid unhealthy choices, like eating junk food. Your family will start to see the difference in the way healthy food makes them feel, giving them the energy they need to walk or run. And people who get exercise sleep better. What's not to love?

When you talk to your family about the event, be sure to talk about how it's fun; not something they *have* to do!

Chapter 6: Self-Improvement

151. Teach yourself to be a good public speaker

This would have to be one of my biggest fears and I know I'm not alone. I don't have any practical advice, but I've heard good things about _Toastmasters_, which is a global organization that helps people to be better communicators, leaders and public speakers.

152. Do something out of your comfort zone

Choose one thing to do over the course of 30 days or write down 30 smaller things to do each day to get yourself out of your comfort zone. If you're stuck for ideas, get someone who knows you well to come up with some suggestions for you.

153. Celebrate small accomplishments

Break big goals into small manageable pieces, enjoy the whole process and celebrate every small accomplishment. This could be something as little as taking a minute out of your day before you go to bed, reflecting on your greatest small accomplishment for the day and feeling grateful.

154. Start that project you've been meaning to do for ages

You can make excuses, but I'm sure there's something you could do right now to make a start on your project, even if it's as simple as sending an email or writing down one thing you can do now to move you forwards in your project.

156. Write down nagging thoughts on paper and thrown them away

At the end of each day, if there's anything on your mind, just write it down on a piece of paper, tear it up and let it go. It might not solve everything but it could help to ease your mind a bit. This is something I often do and find it really helpful.

157. Write a letter to your future self

What advice would you give to yourself in five, 10 or 15 years to come? I've still got some letters that were written from my younger self which are really lovely to read. For example, when I was seven, I wrote a letter advising my future self not to smoke, which I listened to.

You can do this one at any age. Write a sentence a day, then place it in an envelope to read in the future.

158. Keep a thought journal

If the average person has thousands of thoughts a day, what do you spend your time thinking about? If your thoughts shape your beliefs and actions, what could you do today to change what you think about? You won't capture all your thoughts in a journal, but it might help tame your monkey mind and make you more aware of what's going on in your head all day.

159. Keep a diary or journal

Save moments of your life to look back on and reflect in years to come. Write down your thoughts, dreams, or the things that have happened to you today. Draw, write poems or collect memorabilia to glue in.

160. Create a new daily routine for yourself

Wake up at a new time. Eat lunch away from your desk. Spend longer eating breakfast. You don't need to do loads of things here — just pick something and see how it feels.

161. Start a happiness journal

Write down one thing every day that made you smile. It could be moments that are personal to you, things you observe or reflections on happiness in general. In times to come, you can look back on what you've written to help lift your spirits.

162. Learn to read body language

A lot of us are able to read people to some extent, but what else might you learn if you spent a month learning all you can about body language?

163. Plan your outfits the day before

If you spend ages getting ready, this one might help. It might also allow you to think more creatively as you'll have the time to experiment teaming new items together. I did this while I was in college for a bit. It's probably one of the few times in my life when people used to consistently compliment me on my clothes.

164. Be neat and tidy

If you consistently leave loads of washing up in the sink, crumbs on work surfaces, and your house is always messy, try being tidy and more organized for a month and see how it feels. If you feel you don't have the time, start by giving everything a really good clean and take it from there.

165. Develop your common sense and ability to plan ahead

Sometimes with little tasks, I'll make things harder for myself by taking the long way around because I hadn't properly thought about it, but hopefully I'm getting a bit better with this one. If this is an issue, give yourself time to come up with plans rather than rushing ahead, and put more thought into your actions.

166. Be totally honest — so no lying for 30 days

This one might be harder than you think, but it's a good one to observe — just so you can see how often you usually lie. Even if you don't tell big lies, how often do you tell the truth when people ask you how you are, or what about telling the truth to yourself?

167. Create affirmations for your life

You could do this on your way to work, during breaks or when you're waiting in queues. Some people love self-affirmations like me. Read more about how to create affirmations here.

168. Write down a positive thought first thing in the morning

Keep a notebook and pen by the side of your bed and start your day by writing down one positive thought. If you consistently wake up and feel groggy or grumpy about the day ahead, you could see if this makes a difference. A positive thought could also be something you're grateful for — anything that sets your day off to a good start. You just have to mean what you say.

169. Write down ideas for accomplishing a long-term goal

What have you always wanted to do but never have? Give yourself a month to come up with ideas and a small action plan. When you've written down enough things, is there one thing that stands out as being more important than the rest? Start accomplishing your goal by doing this thing first.

170. Do one thing each day that makes you feel inspired

Listen to a song that inspires you, watch a TED talk, be around people you love...select a few things to do over the course of a month or write a list of 30 different things that make you feel inspired each day and put them into action.

171. Spend each day being as 'present' as possible

It might feel boring at first, so you might want to build up to this by practicing being truly present for 30 minutes every day at first. Your key here is to be fully present when you do the tasks that normally send you into autopilot.

172. Decide to become a master at something

In the book *Outliers: The Story of Success*, the author suggests it takes 10,000 hours to become a master at something. However, the following article, *The 10,000 rule is wrong. How to really master a skill,* suggests otherwise. Perhaps you could find out firsthand how long it takes to become a master at something. It will probably take you longer than 30 days, but this could be the start and it might help you prioritize what's most important to you in your life.

173. Develop your introverted or extroverted side

Be comfortable in your own company, learn to listen to others more, and focus on your inner world for a bit. Or spend more time with people who inspire you and make you feel energized just by talking with them. I loved reading *Quiet: The Power of Introverts in a World That Can't Stop Talking*

174. Bring more variety into your life

When I look back on the times in my life where I was doing more new things, I perceive that period of time to have been longer than it was. When I have no variety for a while, time just seems to speed up and the days just merge into one. Make an effort each day to introduce one small thing that's different from your everyday routine. Write out 30 things using your 30 day challenge planner chart and put them into action.

175. Spend time alone

I'm not suggesting you become a hermit, but if you never spend any time alone, consider putting aside at least half an hour every day where you're alone — especially if this is something you never do. How does it make you feel?

176. Do nothing for 30 minutes a day

If you're someone who finds it hard to switch off and relax, make a real effort to do nothing for a short period each day. We live in an illusion where we think the more we do, the more we'll get done, but we have to unwind sometimes too.

177. Trust your intuition and listen to your heart

We live in a time where logic and our minds often overrule our hearts and inner voice. Spend 30 days, really making an effort to listen to what your inner self is saying to you in your everyday life. Record your thoughts in a journal.

178. Work on creating a positive self- image

We live in a world that often makes women feel inadequate about their bodies. This is a bit of a vague one I know, and could well take longer than a month, but you could start with little things such as ditching magazines that make you feel bad and doing other small things that are kind to yourself. It could even be as simple as limiting the amount of negative self talk you might have towards your body.

179. Ditch gossip magazines

I'm not saying they're evil, but if you consume celebrity gossip daily, experiment going cold turkey on it for a month and see how you feel afterwards. What else could you read or learn instead?

180. Hold yourself well

You don't need to sit rigidly straight — just feel relaxed and comfortable with yourself. After I've done yoga and meditation, I feel I can move a lot more freely, as if I'm somehow lighter on my feet and carrying less baggage. Holding yourself well, just means being comfortable with yourself and your body.

Chapter 7: Organization

181. The wallet and/or purse

If you're like me, the dreaded "black bag" seems to collect everything from goldfish (not real goldfish, the crackers) to nail polish, to bills, to gum, mints and everything else under the sun! The first task is to get rid of the crap in the bag. Spend 15-30 minutes cleaning out your bag or purse. Here are some basic guidelines:

- Remove everything and vacuum out the bag

- Organize or toss paperwork and receipts

- Replace only with the bare necessities. 1 pen, 1 chapstick, wallet, phone.

182. The Papers

If you are like me, you probably have a pile of paperwork, homework, and/or bills collecting on your kitchen counter or table. Go through bills, receipts and other paperwork, and toss or shred accordingly anything you don't need. Sort whatever is left over into its proper location.

183. Front entryway and closet

Donate any coats, shoes, accessories that you no longer use. If you are short on space, put items that are out of season into storage somewhere else.

184. Cleaning Supplies

Go through your cleaning supplies {wherever they may be!} and get rid of all of those products that you don't use. Try to use multipurpose cleaners or green cleaning products whenever possible. If you have multiple partially filled bottles of the same product, combine them into one bottle. Toss any old rags or cloths that are at the end of their use.

185. The Fridge and Freezer

Remove all items that are expired or you will not use. Minimize packaging if possible to save space.

186. The Pantry

Toss all items that are expired and get rid of anything that you know you will not use. Don't forget to go through your spices too! Place items that will be expiring soon towards the front.

187. The Kitchen Cabinets

Look for any items you do not use or have room for. Ensure that all Tupperware has matching lids and eliminate as many unnecessary gadgets, cookbooks, and duplicate utensils that you can.

188. The Medicine Cabinets

Medicine is actually best stored outside of the bathroom in a cool, dry place out of the reach of children. Go through all medications and look for items that are expired or that you no longer need. Return expired medications to your local pharmacy for proper disposal.

189. The Dining Area

Commit to keeping your table clutter free. Find storage solutions for all items that frequently find their way to the table. Donate any dishes, serving ware, or other items that you do not use.

190. The Entertainment Area

Make sure all CDs, DVDs etc are in their proper cases and evaluate what you really will use. Music and videos are so easily accessible through our computers and mobile devices, that your CDs and DVDs may be a thing of the past.

191. Magazines and Books

Let go of your magazine hoarding and get rid of any outdated editions. Cut out pages that you would like to keep and sort into a filing system. Recycle or donate old books that you will no longer read and sort the rest in a logical order.

192. The Junk Drawer

Get rid of everything that is not needed. If you have time, use inexpensive plastic containers to store similar items together. Put items that belong elsewhere away.

193. The Desk

File away any needed paperwork and shred remaining papers. Sort smaller office supplies and only keep products that you use. Get rid of those 2014 calendars!

194. Bathroom Cabinets

Go through all beauty products and keep only what you really use. Do you really need all of those hotel shampoo bottles?

195. The Linen Closet

Donate any linens that you no longer use that are still in good condition. Toss any items that are really dingy or have holes.

196. Makeup

Toss anything that is expired, cracked or no longer your style. Pick your favorites and get rid of those other 10 lipstick tubes that you never wear! To find out more about the recommended shelf-life for various make-up, check out this post on **how to organize your makeup**.

197. Jewelry

Sort through all of your jewelry and decide what items you still wear. Donate or toss the rest! If anything you would like to keep needs cleaning or repairs, put them aside to take care of as soon as you can.

198. The Bedroom Closet

Sort through all clothing and ask yourself if you would still buy it today. If not, it is time for it to go!

199. Sock and Underwear Drawer

Go through all of those socks and underwear. Make sure you have matching socks with no holes and only keep what you still wear.

200. The Nightstand

Clear off table top and sort through drawers keeping only what you would need before bed or during the night.

201. Toys

This is always a fun one. Sort through toys to see what your kids still use {and have your kids help out on this one if they are old enough}. Check to see that toys have all parts and are in working order before donating or selling. Toss the rest!

202. Kids Closet

Check to see what clothes still fit and donate the old ones or sort them into a labeled storage bin if you are saving them for younger children.

203. Craft Area

Be ruthless and really evaluate what items you still need and use. Schools will often take extra supplies that you are looking to get rid of.

204. The Laundry Room

Sort through bins and toss any laundry products that are old or not used. Toss any unpaired socks that are hanging around. I'm not quite sure how we ended up with a whole bin full of mismatched socks, but it happened!

205. The Basement

Chances are this is one of the biggest source of clutter. Set a timer for 30-60 minutes and try to get rid of as many items as possible. Use large storage totes to store seasonal items together.

206. The Garage

This one is also a big clutter offender. Again, set a timer and collect as many items as you can that you no longer use or need.

207. The Car

Grab two bags – one for garbage and one for anything that needs to go back in the house. Put everything away in its proper place that you bring back into the house

208. De-clutter the digital crap

Each day, work on something to clean up your digital clutter. Do you have so many contacts on your iPhone that you don't even know where half of them came from? Do you have thousands of pictures that you could care less about? It's time to minimize your digital clutter!

209. Delete Apps

Delete Apps that you don't need. Chances are you've accumulated way too many!

210. Figure out the areas in your life you can simplify

Start with your bedroom for example. Do you have too many blankets, pillows, and clothes lying around? Start by clearing this area of your home. Perhaps limit the decor and comforters. Buy a simple yet comfortable mattress that really doesn't need a lot of added items like mattress toppers.

Chapter 8: Productivity

211. Organize your email inbox.

Take a few minutes to delete emails you don't need, or create folders that'll make organization easier.

212. Get a file folder and organize some documents.

For example, break down each file into a category of bills, and file the paper away once each bill is paid. If you ever need it later on, you'll know exactly where to find it.

213. Set your priorities for the day.

Each morning, decide on the top 3-5 things you want to accomplish. Write it down and spend a minute or two reflecting on how you want your day to unfold. By starting your day with clear intentions, you will be focused on accomplishing what you set out to.

213. Make a to do list for the week ahead.

Productivity depends on planning. Though it's tempting to write a to-do list of daily tasks first thing in the morning, you'll get through that list more efficiently if you write it up a day ahead. That gives you time to mentally prepare for each task and waste less time getting it done

214. Keep track of your activities

See how long each of them take. See if you can save yourself time by eliminating steps.

215. Wake up earlier

Waking early is a habit shared by many of the world's most successful people - and with good reason. Getting up early adds time to get some of the day's most important tasks out of the way and allows you to start working while your mind is alert and refreshed. Those early hours can also be used for exercise, meditation or other healthy things that can often be forgotten in the press of a busy day.

216. Silence Your Phone

Ringing phones and text notifications interrupt concentration and can distract you from the task at hand. When you're working through your to-do list, turn off your phone or set it to silent. Add a time to your schedule for returning calls and messages, and stick to it unless there's an emergency.

217. Create a Workspace You Love

Research on productivity reveals that people are more energized and productive when they're working in a space filled with colors and things that make them feel good. Whether you share an office with others, or you're carving out a workspace in the corner of your bedroom, take time to add good lighting, fill a wall with prints or posters, or arrange your desk just the way you like it.

218. Find an Ergonomic Chair

Many people spend most of their workday sitting - but sitting in an uncomfortable chair can affect both your concentration and your health. Finding an ergonomic chair that's the right height and supports your back and legs can reduce physical distraction, improve your mood and enhance your productivity.

219. De-Clutter Your Workspace

Some studies on productivity suggest that a cluttered work area actually increases stress, hinders concentration and drains your energy. When your desk is a mess, it's harder to find things you need and the overall look is hardly professional. Take a few minutes to tidy up and clear your workspace at the end of the day, or before you start work in the morning, for an easy way to boost productivity.

220. Play Upbeat Music

The relationship of music to productivity has been the subject of intense study, but research suggests that playing upbeat music, rather than soothing, slow tunes, can boost energy and stimulate alertness. In some studies, people worked faster when listening to fast music with a driving beat. This kind of music can also make people happier and more willing to engage with others, so adding an upbeat playlist to your workday can be a simple and fun way to encourage productivity.

221. Drink Enough Water

Dehydration can impair energy and concentration. Drinking enough water - or other fluids - can help improve your focus and keep your body functioning well. Swig cold water or iced tea for an instant wake-up if you're feeling sluggish at your desk.

222. Keep an Agenda with Daily Tasks

It takes more than a daily to-do list to keep track of all the things you need to accomplish, and it's easy to miss less important tasks. Keeping an agenda that's inspired by your big goals lets you schedule in all the jobs that need to get done, and reminds you why they should be done to further your long-term plans.

223. Sort Tasks by Impact and Effort

If you're faced with a lot of tasks to do, setting priorities is essential to getting things done. One way to do that is to sort tasks according to the impact they're likely to have on your goals, versus the effort it takes to get them done. A relatively minor job could have a major effect - or vice versa. Organizing your tasks in this way can save time and avoid spending energy on things that don't yield much return.

224. Set Realistic Deadlines

Deadlines can be intimidating, but they provide a framework for getting things done. Establish deadlines that are realistic and manageable, given the task at hand and the time available. Build in some flexibility for dealing with unexpected problems that could slow you down.

225. Set Goals for the Day, Month and Year

Goals become more achievable when they're broken down into manageable steps. Decide on your big goals for the year, and then set the smaller daily and monthly goals that will lead to completing the yearly plan. Add

these goals to your agendas and to-do lists to keep
them in mind.

226. Focus on One Thing at a Time

Though it may seem that multitasking saves time and
gets more done, productivity studies reveal that just the
opposite is true. The human brain is organized to focus
on one thing at a time, so dealing with multiple tasks
and processing input from many sources at the same
time reduces efficiency and limits your ability to retain
information. What's more, some research suggests that
habitual multitasking may actually reduce your IQ.

227. Plan Breaks

The traditional "nose to the grindstone" approach leads
to burnout and can harm your health. Build short breaks
into your workday to stretch, take a short walk, drink
some water or even exercise for 10 minutes or so. You'll
return to your task refreshed and ready to concentrate.

228. Knock out Your Biggest Task First

Prioritizing can be a challenge if you have a lot of jobs to
do, but putting your biggest task at the top of your to-
do list and getting it done clears space for other things.
It also gives a feeling of accomplishment that sets the
tone for the whole day.

229. Set High Priority Tasks During Your "Peak Hours"

Everyone has a period when they're working at their peak - alert, energized and focused. Whether your "peak hours" are early in the morning, late at night or somewhere in between, use those hours to take care of the most important tasks on your agenda.

230. Work on Delegating Tasks

If you're feeling overwhelmed with too many things to do, consider which tasks, at work or at home, you can delegate to someone else. Make a list of all the jobs that need to be done in a day and decide which ones can be done by a family member or other helper.

231. Work in Intervals and Time Yourself

For many people, working in timed intervals rather than long stretches is a way to improve efficiency and concentration. Set timers or alerts to help pace tasks and remind you to take a break to move around and re-focus.

232. Outsource

Along with delegating tasks to others, outsourcing work related jobs to professionals in those areas can save you time and money. Even getting help for household chores can free your time for doing the tasks that only you can do. If there's anything someone can do better than you can, send that task their way - whether it's taking care of your accounting or cleaning the garage.

233. Designate a Time for Answering Emails

Constantly checking and answering email can consume a lot of productive work time. Turn off email notifications while you're working and schedule a specific time in your workday to answer the ones that are important.

234. Unsubscribe From Distracting Emails

Along with important emails, your inbox may be filled with a variety of distracting notices from lists you've subscribed to. Clean up your email by unsubscribing from any emails that aren't relevant to your goals and interests, or send them to a separate folder to read later.

235. Look for Tools to Improve Your Workflow

If certain areas of your workflow aren't moving as smoothly as you'd like, look for new tools to help. From messaging and meeting apps to schedulers, planners and productivity software, new business tools can save you time and support your long-term goals.

236. Minimize Meeting Time

Meetings may be necessary, but if they're not managed well, they can consume too much productive time. Consider "standing meetings" in which no one sits down, or virtual check-ins and chats with an in-office messaging and team management app.

237. Learn to Say No

Along with delegating and outsourcing tasks to others, learn to say no when you need to. Taking on too many tasks and giving up too much of your time to meet others' needs creates stress and derails your own goals. Don't feel comfortable with saying no? Consider a course or book on setting boundaries to help you get the hang of it.

238. Designate a Break for Social Media

Although social media can be both social and business related, checking your accounts throughout the day consumes work time and affects your concentration. Choose a time such as lunch or an afternoon break to catch up on social media and avoid distractions during work time. If you need help staying away from those distracting sites, consider tools like Leechblock or Nanny - browser extensions that allow you to block specific sites for certain periods of time.

239. Use Your Commute Time

For many people, commuting is a regular part of the workday, and that time can be used for minor work tasks such as checking and answering emails and phone calls, or catching up on reading and research. Consider investing in devices and apps that can help you make your commute time more productive.

240. Exercise Daily

Regular exercise has a long list of well-documented benefits for both the body and mind, and adding daily exercise to your routine can also boost productivity and counter the effects of long periods spent sitting. You don't have to put in long hours at the gym to see the benefits, either. Build exercise into your workday by stretching during breaks, taking a walk at lunch or after work, or using the stairs rather than the elevator.

Chapter 9: Personal Finance

Have you added your monthly income and compared to your monthly expenses and noticed a gap (not where you have more money left over)? If so, you are not alone. Try these 30 day challenges to get finances in check.

241. For 30 days, make all meals at home

The idea here is to take advantage of the fact that cooking at home is far less expensive than eating at a restaurant or consuming delivery food or takeout. It's just cheaper to make food yourself.

The thing that keeps people from jumping on board with this is that cooking is often perceived as difficult and time consuming. Often, people eat prepared food because they're either intimidated by cooking or intimidated by the cleanup.

Committing to this challenge lets you experience the financial savings, as well as, honing your cooking skills. It's about saving money, sure, but it's also about building skills in the kitchen and learning that it's not really that hard to prepare dishes that you like.

242. For 30 days, buy no brand name items

The goal is to introduce you to the store brand version of many products and save money.

There are two exceptions to this challenge. One, if you need an item and the only version is name brand, you can still buy the name brand. Two, if you are making a major planned purchase that you have done the research on.   This challenge pertains to ordinary purchases like groceries and household supplies.

242. For 30 days, don't use credit cards

This one will be hard for those of you (that was me) that buy everything on credit and pay it off (hopefully) at the end of the month.

While normally that's a great strategy, psychologically we spend more money when we use plastic versus when we pay with cash.

By ditching your credit cards for a month, you'll force yourself to use cash (yes, that funky green paper you never see anymore) and start to physically see your money leave your hands as you buy things.

One of the best things about cash is that it's finite. Meaning, once it's gone, it's gone. Take a page out of Dave Ramsey's envelope system method and budget all of your major categories into physical envelopes.

Things like your debt payments, rent, and utilities don't have to be done with cash, but anything that you'll actually be buying should. So groceries and gas will all be cash this month

243. For 30 days, sell or get rid of one item from your closet each day

Many of us have closets in our home that are filled to the brim with stuff – half forgotten or completely forgotten purchases and gifts that were placed in there with the best of intentions of getting around to it someday, but the fact is that someday isn't coming. They're just not things that are a part of your daily life.

The end result for many people is that they have shelves and racks in their closet full of things that they've barely used and are likely never going to use, put in there with good intentions but a lack of time and opportunity.

All of that stuff consumes storage space in your home. The items stored in there are things that someone else might actually put to some kind of productive use.

Perhaps even more important, all of the items stored in there have some amount of secondhand value, which means you can turn them into money in your pocket or charitable gifts for a deduction on your taxes or simply give them to someone because it will make their day.

The challenge is for the next 30 days, dig into your closet and pull out one item each day to sell or to give away. If you're going to sell it, head over to Craigslist or a local Facebook group or eBay or Amazon Marketplace and list it. If you're going to give it away, figure out a friend or a charity that could really use it and unload it there.

The goal is to remove 30 things from your life, whether it's articles of clothing or books or games or something else entirely. Not only will it clear out some space in your home, it will also clear out space in your mind, while also producing some extra cash or goodwill.

244. For 30 days, keep your thermostat five degrees cooler

This is a great challenge during the winter months; for the summer months, shoot for keeping your thermostat five degrees above normal.

In either case, the goal here is to keep your air conditioning or your furnace from running nearly as much for a month, which will save a lot on seasonal heating and cooling costs and it will put money straight in your pocket.

This challenge may require you to push yourself into find strategies for making those new heating and cooling settings work for you.

In the winter, you might want to try things like wearing a sweatshirt and thick socks around the house or running the ceiling fans in a direction so that they pull air upwards rather than blowing it downwards. In the summer, you might try opening the windows and wearing minimal clothing inside and making sure the ceiling fans are all blowing downwards. There are lots of strategies for both seasons to make the temperature more tolerable.

Even if you end up deciding, at the end of the challenge, that a particular temperature is too extreme, you'll probably find that your original setting is probably unnecessary, too, and you'll end up at a happy point somewhere in the middle – something that you now feel completely comfortable with that also results in lower heating and cooling bills.

245. For 30 days, make your morning coffee at home and take it with you in a travel mug.

This is surprisingly easy to do, even if you don't have a coffee maker at home. (If you do, obviously, just brew a couple of cups or a pot before you leave the house and fill up a travel mug to go.)

If you don't have a coffee pot, don't sweat it – just get a simple cold brew coffee maker like this one and start making it in your fridge with ease. All you do is put some coffee grinds in the filtered portion, fill it up with water, and let it sit overnight. The coffee's ready to go in the morning and you just heat it up in the microwave as you wish.

You can try a bunch of different additives and sweeteners to get it just how you like it each morning. Trust me, the cost of buying a few bottles of sweetener and a bag of ground coffee is far less over the course of a month than the cost of buying coffee every day at the coffee shop.

If you can find a mix that you like, then let it become a permanent replacement. The ongoing cost of making your own coffee at home versus buying a big cup at a coffee shop every morning isn't even comparable!

246. For 30 days, don't purchase unnecessary items

Over the course of 30 days, don't buy anything that's not something you need for basic living. Buy the basic food you need, buy store brand household items as needed, and cover your bills.

Instead of starting off nice and slow, you're going to do something to shock your financial system. You're going to stop spending money on anything that isn't an absolute necessity!

Be aggressive with your decisions—don't let yourself off the hook. For example, you might think something like clothes, bed linens, and haircuts are needs. But in reality, you can survive without them!

247. For 30 days, track every dime you spend

Keep a little pocket notebook with you and every time you spend even a penny, you write it down in that notebook for 30 full days. Everything. If you spend a dollar in a vending machine, write it down. If you swipe your credit card to buy a sandwich, write it down. Write everything down. Stick receipts in there for every swipe you make – grocery receipts, gas receipts, everything.

What does this do? First of all, it will give you just a moment's pause with every purchase and will nudge you just a little against silly and unnecessary ones. That's a valuable nudge to have in your life.

The second benefit is a bigger one, though. At the end of the month, you can take all of that info – along with credit card and bank statements to back it up and fill in blanks – and group all of those purchases together however you like.

You can – and should – parse grocery receipts and separate things into sensible categories, like necessary food and frivolous food, necessary household items and frivolous household items. Do this for everything. Make as many categories as you can, but try to make ones that separate needs from wants and impulses.

Then, when you've separated everything, total each grouping and see where your money went.

The thing to remember here is that it's not a problem that you have some frivolous expenses, but the sheer amount that's the problem. If you're shocked by the number, you should be, and you should use that experience as a driver for shaping your future spending habits.

248. Learn how to read your pay stub

It's time to learn how to read one of the most important financial documents that you are most likely ignoring. By breaking down what's on your pay stub, not only will you see where your money is going, but you will also learn about pre-tax savings, which will hopefully encourage you to take advantage of all the ways you can lower your tax bill. Learn how to read your paystub here.

249. Sell your old crap

Spend 30 days sorting through things in your life that you no longer need or use. Sell old clothes on eBay. Sell old CDs, DVDs and other household items you no longer want or need.

250. Double what you save each day

You could start with a really small amount such as one pound or a penny and then the next day save two pounds, on the third day four, and so on. Then at the end of the month either save it or treat yourself.

251. Put your pennies in a jar

You'll be more likely to find loose change if you do this. For example, I spotted two pound coins on the street this morning.

252. Start saving 10% of your income and love doing it

This one has helped me to save a lot more than I usually would since I started doing it, but I understand it's not for everyone. What I will say, is that no matter how much you're earning, it adds up and at the time, you really don't feel like you're missing out on the money.

253. Sell 30 things you don't need, use or wear anymore and see how much money you make at the end of the month

Most of us collect things we never use and allow them to gather dust. Spend a month clearing out all the things you never use that might be worth something.

254. Read yourself rich with these books

There are three books which have greatly influenced my financial mindset:

- <u>Rich Dad Poor Dad: What the Rich Teach Their Kids About Money That the Poor and Middle Class Do Not!</u> by Robert Kivosaki. I read this book when I was in my early 40's and once again now that I'm in my late 40's. Robert Kivosaki's two dads offered him the choice of contrasting points of view. One dad was a highly educated and intelligent man and the other was an entrepreneur who never finished eighth grade. Guess who was the richer of the two!

- <u>The Millionaire Next Door: The Surprising Secrets of America's Wealthy</u> by Thomas J. Stanley. This book is based on 20 years of research on America's self-made millionaires. The book reveals the traits of the affluent: the mindset, the education, the choice of spouse, the clothes they wear, the kind of businesses they run, etc.

- <u>Secrets of the Millionaire Mind: Mastering the Inner Game of Wealth</u> by T. Harv Eker. Harv offers concrete ideas on how to re-program your financial blueprint with accelerated learning techniques and daily declarations.

255. Cut unnecessary subscriptions

Today, evaluate the memberships or subscriptions you pay for. Many individuals and families have subscriptions to magazines, television, apps, and movie streaming services.. not to mention gyms, clubs, online gaming services.

Chances are good, you're paying for a membership that you're probably not using each month. Cancel it now!

If you cancel just 3 memberships that cost $10 per month, you're saving $360 a year.

Tip: I've heard good things about the app <u>Hiatus</u> which helps you manage your recurring subscriptions *but haven't personally used it myself yet.

256. Invest your change and let it grow

If you've tried going back to using cash for everyday purchases and found it just isn't working like the ease of a credit card, then today's task is to set yourself up with change investing. I use and love the <u>Acorns App</u> because it will round my purchases up when I use my credit or debit card and invest the spare change. Over time those investments have grown without me thinking about them and I get a little new found wealth each month.

257. Earn a Minimum of $200 through a Side Hustle

Over the next 30 days set the goal of earning an additional $200 outside your 9-5 career. Walk dogs with Rover, drive with Uber, freelance on Upwork, etc. Get some ideas for side hustles with 100+ Side Hustle Ideas (Almost) Anyone Can Do.

258. Download cash back and promo code apps to get the most of your money.

If you plan on shopping, why not get cash back for your efforts? Here are a few ideas:

- Ebates – get $10 when you spend $25 shopping online

- Ibotta – get $10 as a welcome for grocery shopping online

- Retail-me-not – coupon codes

- Cartwheel – Target shopping

259. Shop smart with lists and coupons

We have talked about the elimination of unnecessary spending and the reduction of needed spending, and now we want to talk about necessary spending.

Commit to creating a shopping list for your next trip to the grocery or drug store. When you make a list, only include items that are necessary. After you make your list, do a search for coupons. A good list can go a long way in helping you keep your shopping in check. When you go to the store, stick to your list.

260. Get to know your monthly expenses

No matter the income level, financial success comes from consistently living below one's means.

Today we are laying the groundwork for becoming a better spender. By reviewing our monthly expenses, you will get a sense of the "big picture".   It will also get you the information you need to build our budget.

261. Build a budget

A budget provides us the input we need to manage our income, track expenses, improve our cash flow, pay off debt and contribute to a savings plan. Create a budget based on your current income and expenses by reviewing your fixed monthly expenses, bank statements, and credit card statements for the last 30 days.   Here is a link to a simple Microsoft budget template that has over 3.4 million downloads. This will help you identify certain areas in which you can make cuts if necessary. For example if your monthly dry cleaning expenses are $125 but you really only have $75 to allocate to this you can see if you need to find a new dry cleaner or take more expensive items to the cleaners less often.

262. Identify recurring expenses

Write down expenses that you know you incur each month. Divide into two categories: essential and non-essential. Include rent/mortgage, car payment, electric and gas, daycare, groceries, etc on the essentials side. Include restaurants, cable, and other discretionary spending on the nonessential side. Add up the total expense. Hopefully your total expenses are less than your total income. If they aren't, consider cutting out some of the expenses on the nonessential side today.

263. Examine your health benefits

Request a copy of your benefits package. Determine if moving to a higher deductible, lower premium plan may benefit you. Also consider mixing and matching health coverage. You may find that your spouse's company has cheaper dental coverage while yours offers better medical. Just be sure to choose a plan that fits your needs. A cheaper plan that offers higher co-pays may not be your best bet if you know your children often need to see their doc. Also make sure to account for higher deductibles in your emergency fund, if you decide to go that route.

264. Reduce your insurance

Take a look at your homeowners/renters and car insurance. First speak to your current provider and see if there's a way to lower your rate. You might be able to increase your deductible (be sure to account for that in your emergency fund), bundle policies or get a loyalty discount. Then shop around and see if any other companies can beat that lower rate. Before you make your calls, see if there is anything else you can do to reduce your risk and therefore your cost.

265. Cut back your cell phone bill

Cutting your recurring bills, especially big ones like cable and cell phone, can make a big dent in your long term savings. Call your current mobile provider to see how you can reduce your bill. Then call around to the competition and see if they can beat the price, just like you did for your insurance yesterday. You might also want to try out these creative hacks for reducing your bill even more.

266. Automate your emergency fund

Most banks offer an option to set up a recurring monthly transfer from your checking account to your savings account. If you're still working on building your emergency fund, set that transfer up to recur monthly. If you're not sure how much money you need in your fund, check out this article.

267. Increase and improve your 401k contributions

Increase your 401(k) contribution to take full advantage of your employer's match. For example, if your employer matches 50% of the first 5% you invest, make sure you're investing at least 5%. Not only is investment in a retirement account going to reduce your tax bill, your employer match is free money, and you should never leave free money on the table. Also take a look at your investment choices. Review the fees and performance for each fund offered and make sure to choose the one that has the right mix of flexibility, risk and reward along with a low fee.

268. Organize and protect your financial records

Getting your financial records in order helps you in your efforts to improve your financial life. Having your financial records organized and in one spot brings clarity and allows you to quickly find documents for reference. Properly protecting your records means you won't be starting over if a fire or other incident leaves you in a bad spot. The bottom line is that having your financial records in order is a sign that you've got your finances in order as well.

Do a search online for a list of financial records you need to keep. See the resources below as well. Take your list and start organizing your financial records into both physical and online folders, as well as a safe. For the longest time, I used a simple accordion style folder and it helped me stay organized.

If you don't have a small, fireproof safe, go buy one. In short, important financial documents you need for the long-term (marriage and birth certificates, will, titles, social security cards, etc.) should be kept in your safe. Remember that video we took on day seven? That should also go in your safe.

All short-term records can be kept in either your physical folders or digitized and kept on your PC, plus some backup service like Dropbox.com

269. Make a will

Talking about making a will is a lot like talking about life insurance. It's necessary, but it might make you uncomfortable. That's okay. As long as you get it done. I have a confession to make. I don't have a will. So today's challenge hits close to home. I'm not going to try to give an excuse. I simple don't have a will, like many of you possibly.

A will is important if you have minor children because it designates where your children will go in the event of you and your spouse's deaths. A will is also important because it dictates how your assets are divided up among your family when you die.

Anyone with significant wealth or a complex family situation should probably go to a lawyer to get their will done. But, as with many things in personal finance, the perfection is the enemy of the good. If you want to make your own will for free or use an online will making program, go for it. For some, their situation is simple enough where this may just work.

If you don't have a will and have kids or assets, then take action today to get a will completed. If you want to use a lawyer, then call today and make an appointment. If you want to use software, then go download it right now.

270. Reduce your tax burden

Taxes are a big part of our financial life. It's hard to avoid them. We pay taxes on our income, our investments, our property, the things we buy, and a bunch of other things.

While you have to pay taxes, there are some things you can do to reduce the amount you pay in taxes, even as your income rises.

You can "shelter" some of your income from taxation or investment by using tax-advantaged accounts, like the 401K, Roth IRA, and 529 Plan.

You can keep your property taxes in check by paying them yourself at the end of the year, as well as by ensuring the municipality is valuing your property correctly.

Finally, you can reduce your income taxes by taking advantage of every deduction and credit that is legally available to you on the federal and state levels. The only way to absolutely ensure this is to learn a little about taxes yourself and then use the help of a CPA and/or tax software to help close the gap.

Look at your income from last year and see if you can shelter more of it. There is still time to fully fund a Traditional IRA and reduce your taxes.

Also, take a look at your property tax situation. Can you reduce your burden there?

Spend some time researching the most common deductions and credits. Reference this list when you are speaking to your CPA or filing your taxes online.

Chapter 10: Happiness

271. Go outside

Exposure to sunlight is thought to increase the brain's release of the body's happiness hormone, serotonin. Even 10 minutes of sun on your skin is associated with boosting mood and helping you feel calm and focused. Just don't forget your SPF!

272. Write down a goal and look at it every day

Pick one thing that you would like to accomplish, write it down on a piece of paper and keep it with you at all times. Every day for the next 30 days, look at your goal first thing in the morning and last thing before bed, more if you can. There's a saying that we become what we think about, so let the things we want to become take over our minds.

273. Say affirmations

The idea is this: whatever it is that you focus your attention on, you're going to feel it, whether it's true or not because our brains can't tell the difference. Affirming the things we want for ourselves, out loud, with meaning and with intention feels awkward, but it has some powerful effects on our subconscious minds.

274. Visualize something you want to achieve

Every day, spend 10 minutes visualizing, in great detail, something that you want to accomplish. Paint the picture in your head, as if you have already achieved it. Engaged all five senses – what you see, hear, feel, taste and smell, and get to that state of accomplishment. It's a fun exercise, and a powerful one too, one that strengthens your mental processes and trains your brain to think with a more creative, action-oriented mindset.

276. Make your bed

Make your bed, first thing, every single morning. It's a simple and mundane task, but if you make your bed every morning, you will have accomplished something right off the bat, and its an important reminder that little things do matter. I highly recommend this incredible commencement speech by a former Navy Seal commander on why the simple act of making your bed can change your life.

277. Practice gratitude

Every morning or evening, think about 3-5 things (or more) that you are grateful for. Write it down and spend some time appreciating those things, so much that the emotions start to well up. It's not enough to think about gratitude, you have to get yourself to a state of gratitude.

278. Pray each morning

You don't have to be religious to pray (studies suggest it has health benefits). Just pray for gratitude, pray for yourself or for other people, for something you wish for, for peace, for health, for an answer or a sign. Whoever you pray to and whatever you pray for, prayer promotes peace, introspection and presence.

279. Watch something funny

Every day, watch a funny video. We don't laugh or smile nearly as much as we should, but it's so important – for positivity, for stress relief, and it even boosts the immune system. And it's the easiest way to feel good, even if it's temporary. <u>Click here</u> for some funny videos to get you chuckling.

280. Write down three positive things about your day

At the end of each day, write down three things that were positive or successful about your day. It forces you to focus on accomplishments and the good things that happened and hopefully put you in a positive mindset.

281. Draw something

Get a sketchbook and spend 10 or 15 minutes drawing, coloring or painting something each day. Draw something if you want to become a better artist, use the creativity muscle of your brain, or simply because it's fun and it's therapeutic.

282. Perform a random act of kindness

Do something nice, selfless and generous for someone else and don't expect anything back. Here are some ideas to get you started.

283. Do something romantic for your partner/spouse

Because it's important to keep the spark alive and show your partner that you appreciate each other. Here is a great list of 50 ways to be romantic for less

286. Practice minimalism

This is an exercise in simplicity. Choose 50 or 75 items (clothes and things) to "live off of" for thirty days.

287. Tell someone you love them or what they mean to you

It's incredibly difficult to be vulnerable to one person. Try reaching out to someone every day with a heartfelt note about how much you love, respect, are grateful for and/or appreciate them. It will teach you to learn to say the things you want to say while you still have the chance to say those things.

288. Give someone a compliment

Say something nice to someone and say it with meaning. It will make you feel better. It will make the other person feel better. Smiles all around!

289. Meditate

Commit to 10 minutes a day for 30 days. It's incredibly difficult to sit in silence and watch your thoughts. Here is a great primer on meditation.

290. Have an early night

Sleep is crucial to our well-being. Deprivation alters activity in some parts of the brain, so if you're sleep deprived, you may have trouble with decision making, problem solving, processing emotions and coping with change. You should be getting at least 7 hours per night, but try going to bed early, not setting an alarm and treating yourself to a lie in.

291. Garden

Plant a seed, buy a plant, or weed your garden. Gardening is often recommended to those with mental health issues, because it ticks so many boxes when it comes to improving the well-being of those who struggle psychologically: it's a form of exercise, it allows you to interact with nature, and it's a meaningful activity as well as a creative outlet. So get those green fingers dirty, and nurture something you can watch grow.

292. Talk to a friend

And make sure they're a positive one! Reach out to people that you love spending time with, making sure that they're the type to leave you feeling inspired, enriched, and connected. By surrounding yourself with inspirational people, you're setting yourself up for a sunnier outlook on life.

293. Work up a sweat

You don't have to be scared of this one. We're not asking for a long, intense workout. It could be a five minute run for a bus, or bowling with friends. Anything that gets your blood pumping is a sure-fire way of boosting your mood.

294. Listen to music

Skip that sad song and turn on something upbeat. Science has shown that as well as boosting your mood, happy music can benefit your body too. Music has an effect on the autonomic nervous system, which is responsible for controlling blood pressure, heartbeat, and the limbic system (responsible for feelings and emotions).

295. Work on a puzzle

Whether it's an old-school jigsaw with missing pieces or a brain training app, puzzles relieve stress by engaging our minds deeply in a lighthearted, 'low-stakes' way. Completing a puzzle also gives us a sense of accomplishment, boosts confidence and increases our self-esteem.

296. Play with an animal

Stroking a pet has been proven to reduce stress and anxiety. Find a furry friend to spend some time with and see if you feel happier after. If you're still in doubt, just ask the people in care homes, hospitals, or disaster areas, receiving affection from specially trained therapy animals.

297. Stop procrastinating

Crossing something off your to do list will give you a sense of accomplishment and relief, especially if you've been putting a task off for ages. It might even motivate you further to do something else you've been delaying for ages and provide you with a sense of relief when it's finally done.

298. Get dressed up

Make yourself look your best for no-one other than yourself. Take control of how you're presenting yourself and put on your favorite dress for that trip to the supermarket.

299. Learn a new skill

New skills boost our self-confidence and sense of worth, while keeping us curious, and, of course, helping us learn how to do something new. Join a choir, learn a language online, and take yourself out of your comfort zone. You'll thank yourself for it later.

300. Treat yourself

Don't be afraid to treat yourself. Whether it's a daily pick me up such as a pastry from your favorite bakery or some savings that you use once a month for something more special, make sure you treat yourself.

Chapter 11: Kindness

301. Give back to the planet

Write out 30 things you can do each day to be kinder to the planet such as picking up litter, not drinking from takeaway coffee cups, planting trees and flowers or volunteering for an environmental charity. You can then spend 30 days implementing them.

302. Give up your seat if you commute by train

In London, people can be really pushy to get on trains when it comes to rush hour. It's always really heartening when someone offers someone their seat when the train is packed full of people.

303. Buy homeless people hot drinks

Buy 30 hot drinks in 30 days or volunteer for a homeless charity.

304. Give a compliment a day

You could really help to make someone's day. Just make sure you're genuine. People can tell when it's fake.

305. Volunteer for a cause you believe in

Work at a hospice, volunteer at a farm or work with the elderly or homeless. You don't even need to volunteer for a charity — how about helping out one of your neighbors?

306. Give people hugs

You don't have to stand out in the street wearing a sign that says free hugs, but you could become more aware of how you hug people you're close to. We can all tell the difference between a heartfelt hug and one that's just for show or good manners. Make it your mission for a month to always hug people like you mean it.

307. Don't check your phone when you're with people

You might not even realize how much you do this one until you make an effort to stop. The people around you, even if they're not close friends or family, will really appreciate it. In a time when we're all glued to our phones, we need human connection more than ever.

308. Speak kindly about people

I love hearing people saying genuinely kind things about others. Next time you feel like you might start to gossip or bad mouth someone, see if you can turn it around and say something constructive instead.

309. Give people your full attention

How many of us really do this? Obviously, don't let people drain your energy, but try making eye contact more, being fully present when people talk to you, and making people feel valued. Every now and again I'll meet someone who's an incredible listener and it'll make me think about how well I listen and how often we get distracted as humans when we're interacting with others. People can sense it when you're really tuned into them — it's a really wonderful gift to give to someone.

310. Thank, tip or give small presents to people who aren't expecting it

We may be accustomed to tip at restaurants, but who else are you grateful for that you wouldn't normally thank? Try to find one person a day and show them that you appreciate the work they're doing.

311. Treat everyone with the same respect

Do you secretly look down on people you think aren't as good as you or suck up to those in a higher position? Even if you think you don't do this, observe your behavior around everyone and make your own mind up.

312. Write out and do 30 different random acts of kindness

These could be simple things like helping someone with their shopping, thanking someone who wouldn't normally be thanked for the work they do or buying someone who needs it a hot drink.

313. Do karma yoga (selfless service) for at least 15 mins a day

Karma yoga is basically doing one good deed a day or selfless action. This could be anything from cleaning floors to serving food or just making people you care about cups of tea.

314. Spend 30 days fundraising for a charity or cause of your choice

Join an existing event or make your own up for a charity that's dear to your heart.

315. Send appreciation notes

Find one thing a day to appreciate and write or send a tweet that shows your gratitude. It could be to a person who has done something nice, a note to someone you love but have taken for granted recently, or it could be completely random like a note left on a window saying 'I appreciate this beautiful view'.

316. Be the one to end gossipy conversations

It starts with one person gossiping about someone, and then someone else in that group agrees or adds their bit, or worse influences everyone else to think the same and then people bond over mutual gossiping, which to me is really wrong. I always respect people who change the subject or end the conversation.

317. Leave food in your garden for birds

Rather than throwing away food scraps, you could give it to the birds — just make sure it's suitable for them to eat. Who doesn't enjoy seeing birds through the kitchen window?

318. Get to know your neighbors

Give yourself a month to get to know more of your neighbors. In big cities like New York, people can live for years in a place without knowing their next-door neighbors' names.

319. Introduce your friends/ acquaintances/ contacts to one another

In your circle of friends, acquaintances and contacts, who could you introduce? Do you know someone who is an expert in their field and someone else who is trying to break into that field? Introduce them. Or just two people you feel would really benefit from knowing one another.

320. See the good in people

This doesn't mean ignoring the undesirable things in others, it just means giving people more of a chance, so you can see more of the good in them.

321. Give away some of your things for free

If you've just cleared out your wardrobe, give away items to friends who you think that piece of clothing would suit. If you're clearing out food cupboards, donate items to a food bank. Could you give away old furniture to a family who might really benefit from it?

322. Be a person of action and words

We all want to hear lovely things and be told how wonderful we are. But these words are empty if there are no actions to back them up. Watch your behavior in your relationships with people and observe your action/word balance.

323. Remember little things people say

I'm always touched when I meet a friend of a friend, and I see them after a half a year or longer and they've remembered certain details from the last conversation we had. It might seem small, but this one will really mean a lot to people.

324. Be humble

If you're obsessed with status and fancy job titles and your ego has become a bit inflated, reflect on being humble for a month. This isn't the same as having low self-esteem.

325. Drop off old blankets and pillows at an animal shelter

Animal shelters and pet rescues are almost always in need of donated supplies for their animals. If you have blankets and towels that you no longer want or need, contact your local animal shelter or animal rescue by phone or in person and ask them when and where to drop off the items.

326. Pay it forward at a drive thru

At a drive through, pay for the car behind's meal or coffee. You could do this at the train station, at a coffee shop – anywhere you like.

327. Pay attention

It's basic courtesy to pay attention when someone is speaking to you. It also shows that you care about them and what they say.   So put everything aside. Avoid multi-tasking. And focus on what they're saying.

If you're having a face-to-face conversation, look into the other person's eyes. Listen to their words. Join their emotions.

In a phone conversation, pay even more attention because you're speaking through a mechanical device.

You must give before you can receive.

328. Have you discovered something that has changed your life?

Share what you know and inspire others to change their lives too!

329. Let someone in when vying for a position in traffic.

Especially in busy metro areas or Southern California, traffic can be very frustrating! Instead of inching ahead, help with the merging process and everyone will speed up together.

330. Spread the kindness!

Let others know you are on a mission to spread kindness and they may just be inspired to do the same!

Chapter 12: Be the Best YOU!

Chapter 12 is a compilation of all the other chapters, but basically it comes down to one thing. Be the best person you can be and here are some challenges to get you started!

331. Find a mentor

What do you want to do with your career or studies? Locate a mentor who can guide you toward your goal. Do your research. Find someone that does what you want to do, and reach out through social networking sites to connect with them and ask questions. Your mentor doesn't even have to work or live in the same place as you.

332. Learn a skill

This suggestion is very broad, but you can cater this goal to an area of your life you would like to improve. For example, you could learn how to create Excel formulas, how to use Photoshop, or how to code in HTML. Or, you could learn how to play an instrument, cook a new dish, knit, or speak a new language.

333. Take pics

Take a picture a day. The picture can be of something as mundane as a water bottle or as cool as one of the 7 Wonders of The World. But seriously, take a picture once per day of the places and things you interact with.

334. Go on a media fast

Sometimes we try so hard to stay connected with all things digital, that we forget to connect with those around us. If a full media fast is too daunting, you can take baby steps. Start by cutting out Facebook or Twitter for a month.

335. Create a thankful list

Sometimes people complete this challenge by listing everything they are thankful for, including the pet goldfish they had when they were a kid. While this is a good way to create a thankful list, I would like to add a twist to it. We can be thankful for things that happen every day, not just in the past. Each day, add an item to the list that is something you are thankful for from that day. This challenge can open your eyes to all the awesome things that happen to you each day. (Side note: If you want supreme happiness as an end goal, I recommend this challenge.)

336. Try New Food

Train your taste buds to like a new kind of food. I am
not a big fan of seafood, but I also haven't eaten it in a
while. For this challenge, I would try different variations
of seafood during the month.

337. Random Acts of Kindness

Perform an act of service each day. It doesn't matter
how big or small. Hold the door for someone, donate
blood, or help someone move. You could even call one
of those "How is my driving?" numbers and report good
driving.

338. Cut out a Bad Habit

Cut out a bad habit over the next 30 days. Some ideas
include smoking, complaining, tardiness, excessive TV
time, impulse shopping, and unnecessary stress. Most
studies conclude that it takes between 21 and 66 days
to form a habit. Even if a habit takes you 66 days to
create, completing a 30-day challenge gets you halfway
there.

339. Exercise

This is another fairly broad challenge. You can take
10,000 steps each day, or even take the stairs wherever

you go (maybe skip the Eiffel Tower on this challenge).
Exercise at least 15 minutes a day with no excuses, and
make an effort to add some extra physical activity to
each day.

340. Thank Someone

You could send a quick Facebook message to a teacher
who made a difference in your life. Even a simple thank
you to someone who held a door open for you counts.
You can even add to this goal by formally thanking 10
people during the month. Either way, you are thanking
people who may have otherwise gone unthanked.

341. Explore your City/State

When planning or dreaming about vacations, most
people don't think about visiting new places within their
own state. Plan a staycation. Go somewhere in your
own city or state you haven't been to before. See a new
local landmark, park, or restaurant.

342. Avoid Negative Language

Avoid words like "can't," "shouldn't," or "don't." People
typically use words like these in an attempt to evade
ownership of a situation. While small, if said enough,
these words can become thought patterns. Instead of "I
can't go," try "I'm sorry. I have another activity going

on." Positive language helps us take control of a situation and better express ourselves.

343. Start a Thought Journal

Have you ever had an great idea or thought and then forgotten it? Was it an amazing business idea? Maybe you made a connection between the theory of relativity and losing weight? Write down all of those awesome ideas and thoughts, even if you think you'll never forget (because you will, unless you write it down. Trust me!).

344. Memorize

Increase your brain strength by memorizing something. Poems might be a good option—you can find poems in different lengths and for different memorizing capabilities very easily. As a bonus, poems can teach you important lessons or cheer you up.

345. Laugh Each Day

Take part in activities that make you laugh. Do funny YouTube cat videos make you laugh? Then watch some! Does hanging out with your family usually result in laughter? Then hang out with your family. Take time to laugh every day for 30 day. You'll be surprised with how much this can boost your mood.

346. Set Goals

So, I stole this exercise from "The Seven Habits of Highly Effective People." What would you want people to say at your funeral? Usually, this exercise results in a list of characteristics like: kind, helpful, smart, etc. This challenge can center on creating 30 individual goals or character traits you would like to develop, or it can be just working on one character trait you would like to improve.

347. Play Brain Games

Exercise your brain with activities like crossword puzzles or Sudoku. They will help you and your brain function at a higher level.

348. Read a Book

Any kind of book—it doesn't matter. Read a fantasy book for fun or a self-help book for ideas on how to improve. Books can relieve stress while increasing vocabulary and intelligence.

349. Wake up Early

There is quite a bit of debate on whether successful people wake up early. This article lists successful people who wake up early, while this article lists successful

people who stay up late. But, you might as well test out
the theory on your own, right? You can do this by
setting your alarm clock a half hour earlier than normal.
If you usually hit the snooze button, try setting several
alarms in succession to ensure you wake up.

350. Create Something

The options for things you could create are limitless.
Grow a Chia Pet or a plant. Make a quilt. Make pottery.
Paint or draw something. Put together a table. Use your
hands to create one or more somethings over 30 days.

351. Be More Charitable

Research a charity that stands for something you
believe in and take part in it. You can start by
performing a simple Google search for causes you are
passionate about. If you like animals, you could
volunteer at an animal shelter. Or, maybe a charity
needs someone to go door to door asking for donations.
Maybe you could volunteer at a hospital. Just choose
one of the many possibilities for charitable work.

352. Research History

Stretch your brain and learn about a period of history,
or a subject that interests you, like: the Declaration of
Independence, the Titanic, World War II, ancient Greek

civilizations, the French Revolution, the origins of Google. The list goes on and on.

353. Save $100

This amount is somewhat arbitrary, and you can change it according to your budget or lifestyle, but the purpose behind this goal is to save. Save $100 by cutting purchases out of your life that aren't necessary. Could you save $100 by not eating out as much? Whatever the amount is, stretch yourself and put some money away in savings.

354. Write your Bucket List

Our moods change from day to day, so I wouldn't be surprised if a bucket list changed from day to day. For this purpose, add at least one item to your bucket list each day. At the end of the month, you will have a list of 30+ awesome things to help you start setting goals.

355. Live Healthier

This one is also pretty broad, but try being healthier for 30 days. This can include cutting out fast food, caffeine, soda, or sugar or even just going on a walk.

356. Watch Ted Talks

TED Talks are pretty awesome, inspirational, and educational. Watch one TED Talk per day. You can start by watching the TED talk about setting 30-day challenges.

357. Set Business Goals

If you are reading this blog you probably own and operate a small business. Set manageable 30-day goals to improve your business. You may want to optimize a page per day on your website or ask for a review once per day. Whatever it is, put your business in a better place by the end of the 30 days.

358. Look for Passive Income

Generate income outside of your normal job. Bonus points if the passive income comes through a passion of yours. For me, that would mean generating additional income through sports, like coaching or selling a sports product.

359. Don't Complain

It's pretty easy to find things to complain about. If you look, it's also pretty easy to find things to be happy about. Complaining, usually, brings about bitterness and unhappiness. And, as you know from this post, that is the opposite of what I want. So a challenge to get rid of unhappiness is right up my alley.

360. The list of possible 30-day challenges is limitless.

Again, you don't have to start with a crazy challenge. Do one challenge and work your way up. Hopefully, this list sparked an idea for a 30-day challenge you are interested in completing. I would love to see what 30-day challenges you are doing and how the process is going. Share your experiences with us in comments on our website iChallengeHub.com or our Facebook Page.

~~The End~~ The Beginning of your 30 Day Challenge

Thank you for reading A Challenge A Day…. 365 30 Day Challenges Ideas to Inspire, Motivate and Change Your Life!

I hope you get everything you want and more from the 30 day challenges you choose to do and that they bring you joy, happiness, more balance, and something to look forward to in your day-to-day life. If you haven't already, don't forget you can download and print out your free 30 day challenge planner chart to help you track and document your progress. Use the link below.

We take requests. Are you interested in a particular 30 day challenge that you don't see here? Send us your request at ichallengehub@gmail.com

If you have enjoyed reading this book, we would be grateful if you would write a review on Amazon sharing your thoughts about the book and/ or how your 30 day challenges are going.

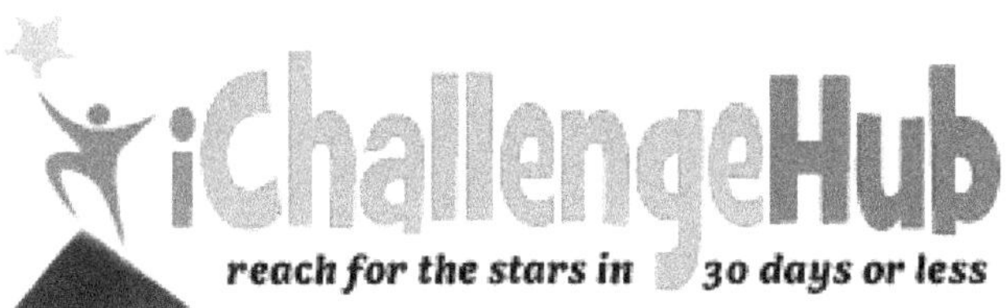

iChallengeHub
reach for the stars in 30 days or less

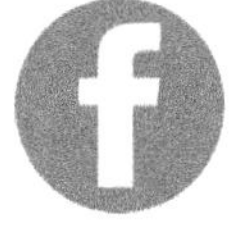
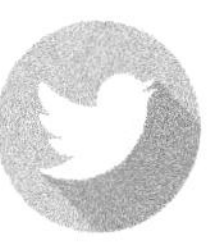

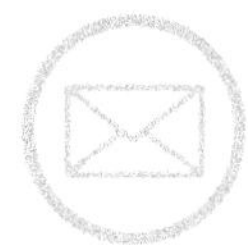